Ophthalmology

AN ILLUSTRATED COLOUR TEXT

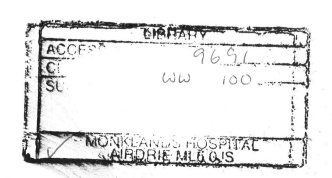

Commissioning Editor: Michael Parkinson
Project Editor: Lynn Watt
Project Controller: Nancy Arnott
Designer: Erik Bigland
Illustration Manager: Bruce Hogarth
Illustrated by: Paul Richardson, Robert Britton

Ophthalmology

SECOND EDITION

AN ILLUSTRATED COLOUR TEXT

MARK BATTERBURY BSc FRCS (Glasg) FRCOphth
Consultant Ophthalmologist, St Paul's Eye Unit,
Royal Liverpool and Broadgreen University Hospitals NHS Trust
Director of Clinical Studies and Honorary Lecturer
Departments of Medicine and Orthoptics
University of Liverpool, Liverpool, UK

BRAD BOWLING FRCSEd(Ophth) FRCOphth
Specialist Registrar, Oxford Eye Hospital
Oxford, UK

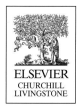

ELSEVIER
CHURCHILL
LIVINGSTONE

EDINBURGH   LONDON   NEW YORK   OXFORD   PHILADELPHIA   ST LOUIS   SYDNEY   TORONTO   2005

ELSEVIER
CHURCHILL
LIVINGSTONE

First edition 1999
Second edition 2005
   Reprinted 2005

ISBN 0 443 07296 5

British Library Cataloguing in Publication Data
A catalogue record for this book is available from the British Library

Library of Congress Cataloguing in Publication Data
A catalogue record for this book is available from the Library of Congress

Note
Medical knowledge is constantly changing. Standard safety precautions must be followed, but as new research and clinical experience broaden our knowledge, changes in treatment and drug therapy may become necessary or appropriate. Readers are advised to check the most current product information provided by the manufacturer of each drug to be administered to verify the recommended dose, the method and duration of administration, and contraindications. It is the responsibility of the practitioner, relying on experience and knowledge of the patient, to determine dosages and the best treatment for each individual patient. Neither the Publisher nor the author assumes any liability for any injury and/or damage to persons or property arising from this publication.

The Publisher

ELSEVIER your source for books, journals and multimedia in the health sciences

www.elsevierhealth.com

Working together to grow libraries in developing countries

www.elsevier.com | www.bookaid.org | www.sabre.org

ELSEVIER   BOOK AID International   Sabre Foundation

The publisher's policy is to use **paper manufactured from sustainable forests**

Printed in China

Preface to first edition

This introductory text to ophthalmology repeats the approach of others in the Illustrated Colour Text series. Double-page spreads combining simple-to-read text, colour illustrations, tables and 'key point' summaries are used to present each topic as a self-contained educational unit.

The contents are divided into four sections. The first contains essential anatomy and physiology, including a novel presentation of the mechanism of human sight, together with an introduction to disease processes and therapy. The second section describes ophthalmic diseases using a traditional anatomically-ordered approach. The third section deals with a collection of special topics, some disease related, others covering clinical management. The final section, presented in an innovative format, is concerned with decision-making in the clinical situation. The reader is presented with scenarios corresponding to the chief clinical problems in ophthalmology. Each scenario can be followed through a number of diagnostic paths via a series of questions and answers. The section may be used for self-assessment following study of the preceding sections or as a practical guide in a clinical setting.

This book is aimed primarily at the medical student, but we believe it will also be useful to orthoptic and optometric students and professionals, to general practitioners and other non-ophthalmic medical practitioners and to nurses.

1999   M.B.
Liverpool and Cardiff   B.B.

Preface to second edition

The text has been extensively revised and updated to correct inaccuracies, to improve clarity and understanding, especially in response to feedback from helpful students, and to keep pace with new developments in ophthalmology. Some of the spreads have been expanded, reflecting the importance to the reader of the subject matter or the new knowledge. We have also added a spread about genetic disease and a database of organisations and information resources.

2004   M.B
Liverpool and Oxford   B.B.

Acknowledgements

Lynn Watt has shown great patience in her efforts to ensure that this second edition was eventually completed and always imparted a reassuring optimism that our tendency to make everything longer would be accommodated somehow. We thank her for her work. We are also grateful to the artists working with Elsevier, and to Jim Killgore for the first edition.

We thank the many people who have helped with the colour photographs, both for this edition and for the first. In particular Ronnie, Steve, Karen and Jerry of the St Paul's Eye Unit Department of Medical Photography; Simon Harding, David Wong, Stephen Kaye, Debbie Broadbent, Paul Hiscott, Peter Wishart, Chris Lloyd, Brian Leatherbarrow, Steve Charles, Peng Khan, Jeremy Butcher, Ian Pearce, Jayashree Sahni and Jack Kanski who kindly provided us with photographs from their own collection.

Colin Willoughby, Lecturer in Ophthalmology at the University of Liverpool and expert in ocular genetics, contributed the genetics spread, giving of his precious time whilst writing up research papers and his MD thesis. Daniel Brotchie, also of the University of Liverpool, allowed us to use the database of resources and organisations that he has painstakingly constructed over several years.

We have been heartened by the many people who have commented favourably on the first edition and have tried to assimilate into this second edition their many suggestions for change and improvement.

Brad Bowling thanks his wife, Suzanne, and son, Edward, for their support and encouragement. Mark Batterbury's family have grown used to the phrase 'I've got to do some book work' when the weekend's activities have to be planned, but their appreciation of the finished product of the first edition helped them be patient and tolerant, for which they are greatly thanked.

Mark Batterbury
Brad Bowling

Contents

Basic Principles

Anatomy and physiology: outer eye

Eyelids

The eyelids (Figs 1 & 2) fulfil two main functions:

- protection of the eyeball
- secretion, distribution and drainage of tears.

Lid movement

The space between the lids is termed the palpebral aperture or fissure. The orbicularis oculi muscle is arranged as a ring of fibres around the palpebral aperture: contraction causes the lids to close. Opening of the lids is principally performed by the levator muscle in the upper lid, though there are some tenuous fibres which act to retract the lower lid. The levator extends from an attachment at the orbital apex to attachments at the tarsal plate and skin (forming a skin crease). The lids are securely attached at either end to the bony orbital margin by the medial and lateral palpebral (or canthal) ligaments. Trauma to the medial ligament causes the lid to flop forward and laterally, impairing function and cosmesis.

Blinking distributes tears across the cornea, which maintains the smooth optical surface of the cornea and displaces debris. There is a brisk protective blink reflex: the afferent limb is the optic, trigeminal (touch) or auditory nerve; the afferent limb is the facial nerve. The eyelashes are also protective.

Skin and appendages

The skin of the eyelids is thin and only loosely attached to the underlying tissues, so that inflammation and bleeding may cause considerable swelling. The semi-rigid tarsal plate lies behind the skin and orbicularis muscle and is lined posteriorly by conjunctiva. It contains the meibomian glands which produce the oily lipid layer of the tear film. These glands are aligned vertically in the tarsal plate and open onto the eyelid margin, where their orifices can be seen. The tarsal plates are continuous peripherally with the orbital septum, a thin but important structural division between the eyelids and the orbit. Along the eyelid margins are the eyelashes anteriorly, the meibomian orifices posteriorly and, at the nasal end, an opening into the tear drainage system (punctum). The grey line, an important landmark in repairing lacerations of the lid margin, is located between the eyelashes and the meibomian orifices.

Innervation

Sensory innervation is from the trigeminal (fifth) cranial nerve, via the ophthalmic division (upper lid) and maxillary division (lower lid). The orbicularis oculi is innervated by the facial (seventh) nerve. A palsy causes an ectropion of the lower lid, but **not** a ptosis. The levator muscle in the upper lid is supplied by the oculomotor (third) nerve. Palsy of **this** nerve does cause a ptosis. Note that all the nerves except the facial nerve reach the lids from within the orbit.

Blood supply and lymphatics

The eyelids are supplied by an extensive network of blood vessels which form an anastomosis between branches

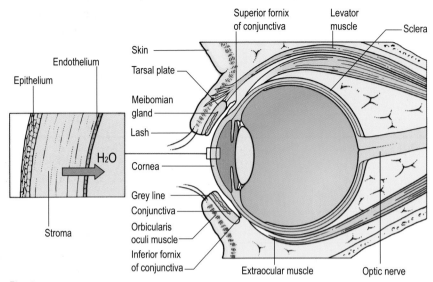

Fig. 1 **Eyelids and eyeball in sagittal section.**

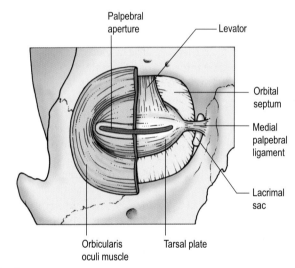

Fig. 2 **Eyelid structure anteriorly** (right eye)**.**

derived from the external carotid artery via the face and from the internal carotid artery via the orbit. This accounts for the excellent healing which follows trauma.

Lymphatic fluid drains into the preauricular and submandibular nodes. Preauricular lymphadenopathy is a useful sign of infective eyelid swelling (especially viral).

Conjunctiva

The conjunctiva is a mucous membrane lining the eyelids and covering the anterior eyeball up to the edge of the cornea. At the upper and lower reflections between eyeball and eyelid the conjunctiva forms two sacs, the superior and inferior fornices (Fig. 1). The conjunctiva is tightly adherent to the lid, loosely attached to the eyeball and free in the fornices. Therefore, inflammation can cause gross swelling of the forniceal and bulbar conjunctiva.

The conjunctiva comprises an epithelium and an underlying stroma. Within the epithelium are goblet cells, which secrete the mucin component of the tear film. Conjunctival glands contribute to the secretion of the aqueous and lipid layers of the tear film.

The conjunctiva facilitates free movement of the eyeball and provides a smooth surface as the lids blink against the cornea.

Sensory innervation is mediated via the ophthalmic division of the trigeminal nerve. Blood comes mostly from the orbit, but anastomoses with the facial system.

The conjunctiva has an important role in the protection of the eye against microorganisms.

Cornea and sclera

Together, the cornea and sclera form a spherical shell which makes up the outer wall of the eyeball. Although the two are very similar in many ways, the corneal structure is uniquely modified to transmit and refract light.

The sclera is principally collagenous, avascular (apart from some vessels on its surface) and relatively acellular. It is tough despite being thin (maximum thickness 1 mm), and it gives attachment to the extraocular muscles. It is perforated posteriorly by the optic nerve, and by sensory and motor nerves and blood vessels to the eyeball. The cornea and sclera merge at the corneal edge (the limbus).

The cornea consists of a stroma sandwiched between a multilayered epithelium and an inner monolayer of endothelial cells. At the centre the cornea is 500 μm thick, increasing to 700 μm at the periphery. It is nevertheless very strong. The stroma comprises 90% of the thickness, and it is a mixture of collagen and extracellular matrix. There are few cells and no blood vessels.

The cornea is exquisitely sensitive to touch (in contrast to the insensitive sclera) through nerve fibres from the ophthalmic division of the trigeminal nerve. These are exposed when the corneal epithelium is lost, causing great pain.

The cornea is avascular, deriving its nutrition by diffusion from blood vessels at the limbus, from the aqueous humour and from the tear film. Limbal ischaemia can lead to peripheral corneal thinning ('melting'), and prevention of oxygen diffusion from the tear film (e.g. by a contact lens) may result in ulceration.

The chief functions of the cornea are protection against invasion of microorganisms into the eye, and the transmission and focusing (refraction) of light.

Refraction of light occurs because of the curved shape of the cornea and its greater refractive index compared with air. The cornea is transparent because of the specialised arrangement of the collagen fibrils within the stroma, which must be kept in a state of relative dehydration. This is achieved by an energy-dependent ion pump in the endothelium (direction of flow is from stroma to anterior chamber).

The epithelium undergoes constant turnover, basal cells replicating, migrating to the surface and then being shed. In contrast, endothelial cells do not divide. This is of great clinical significance, since there is a critical number of endothelial cells below which there is insufficient pump activity to maintain corneal dehydration. In consequence, the cornea swells and loses its transparency, termed corneal decompensation or bullous keratopathy. Common causes of endothelial cell loss include normal ageing and intraocular surgery (including cataract surgery).

Tear production and drainage

Tears comprise water, mucus to bind the tear film to the corneal epithelium and an outer lipid layer to reduce evaporation of the water. Tears also contain some chemicals against microorganisms.

The lacrimal gland secretes most of the aqueous component of the tear film (Fig. 3). It lies in the superotemporal part of the anterior orbit. Its anterior lobe can sometimes be seen in the upper conjunctival fornix. It is innervated by parasympathetic fibres carried by the facial nerve.

Tears collect in a meniscus on the lower lid margin, are spread across the ocular surfaces by blinking, and drain into the superior and inferior puncta at the nasal end of the eyelids. Single canaliculi from each punctum unite in a common canaliculus which ends in the lacrimal sac. This is in a bony fossa crossed anteriorly by the horizontally directed medial palpebral ligament (Fig. 2). Finally, tears pass down the nasolacrimal duct and reach the nasopharyngeal cavity via the inferior meatus. This accounts for the unpleasant taste which follows administration of certain eyedrops.

At birth, the nasolacrimal duct may not be fully developed, causing a watery eye. In most cases, full canalisation occurs within a year. Acquired obstruction of the nasolacrimal duct is a common cause of a watery eye in adults. It may lead to an acute infection of the sac, which manifests as a cellulitic swelling just below the medial palpebral ligament.

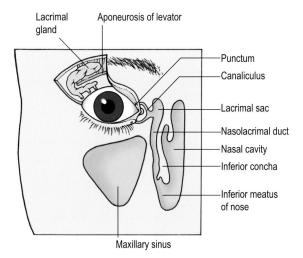

Lacrimal gland
Aponeurosis of levator
Punctum
Canaliculus
Lacrimal sac
Nasolacrimal duct
Nasal cavity
Inferior concha
Inferior meatus of nose
Maxillary sinus

Fig. 3 **Tear production and drainage** (right eye).

> ## Anatomy and physiology: outer eye
>
> ### Eyelids
> - protect the eyeball and distribute tears across the cornea
> - closure by contraction of orbicularis oculi muscle (facial nerve)
> - opening by levator muscle (oculomotor nerve)
> - lid margin comprises a row of lashes in front of a row of meibomian gland orifices separated by the grey line.
>
> ### Conjunctiva
> - a mucous membrane which contributes to tear production and resistance to infection.
>
> ### Cornea
> - a highly specialised tissue
> - main function is refraction and transmission of light
> - structure is an outer epithelium, an avascular hypocellular stroma and a non-replicating endothelial monolayer
> - the endothelium pumps water out of the stroma into the anterior chamber; failure leads to loss of transparency.
>
> ### Tears
> - oily lipid layer secreted by meibomian glands; aqueous layer by lacrimal and conjunctival glands; mucin by conjunctival goblet cells
> - drain into the puncta, then canaliculi, then lacrimal sac, then into nose via nasolacrimal duct.
>
> ### Sensation
> - trigeminal nerve, mostly via the ophthalmic division (maxillary to the lower lid).

Anatomy and physiology: inner eye

The internal ocular structures function primarily to refine the image formed by the cornea, and to convert light energy into electrical energy for image formation by the brain.

Uvea

The uvea comprises the iris and ciliary body anteriorly and the choroid posteriorly (Fig. 1).

Iris

The iris largely consists of connective tissue containing muscle fibres, blood vessels and pigment cells. Its posterior surface is lined by a layer of pigment cells. At its centre is an aperture, the pupil. The chief functions of the iris are to control light entry to the retina and to reduce intraocular light scatter. Pupil dilation is caused by contraction of radial smooth muscle fibres innervated by the sympathetic nervous system. Pupil constriction occurs when a ring of smooth muscle fibres around the pupil contracts. These are innervated by the parasympathetic nervous system (oculomotor nerve).

Iris pigment reduces intraocular light scatter. The amount of iris pigment determines eye 'colour': blue eyes have the least pigment, brown eyes the most.

Ciliary body

The ciliary body (Fig. 1) is a specialised structure uniting the iris with the choroid. It makes aqueous humour and anchors the lens via the zonules, through which it modulates lens convexity.

Anteriorly the inner surface is folded into ciliary processes which are the site of aqueous humour formation. Muscle fibres within the ciliary body contract, causing its inner circumference to reduce. This reduces the tension on the zonules, so that the natural elasticity of the lens causes it to become more convex to focus on near objects. This is called accommodation and is controlled by parasympathetic fibres

in the oculomotor nerve. Relaxation is passive, increasing tension on the zonules so that the lens is pulled flat for distance vision.

The posterior part of the ciliary body merges into the retina at the ora serrata.

Choroid

The choroid, consisting of blood vessels, connective tissue and pigment cells, is sandwiched between the retina and the sclera. It provides oxygen and nutrition to the outer retinal layers. There is a potential space between the choroid and the sclera, which can become filled with blood or serous fluid.

Lens

The discus-like lens (Fig. 1) comprises a mass of long cells known as fibres. At the centre these fibres are compacted into a hard nucleus surrounded by less dense fibres, the cortex. The whole lens is enclosed within an elastic capsule and is deformable for accommodation. Failure of accommodation with ageing (presbyopia) occurs through loss of capsule elasticity and lens deformability.

The lens is relatively dehydrated and its fibres contain special proteins. This is why it is transparent. Cataract occurs when this organisation is disrupted.

Aqueous humour

Aqueous humour fills the anterior and posterior chambers. The anterior chamber is the space between the cornea and the iris. Behind the iris and in front of the lens is the posterior chamber. The two are connected by the pupil.

Formation

The ciliary body forms aqueous humour (or aqueous) by ultrafiltration and active secretion. Its composition is strictly regulated to exclude large proteins and cells, but it does contain glucose, oxygen and amino acids for the cornea and lens. Neural control is via the sympathetic autonomic nervous system (beta receptors).

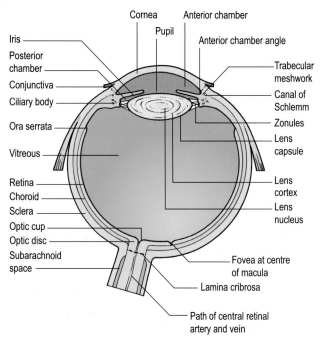

Fig. 1 **Sagittal section of the eye** (right eye).

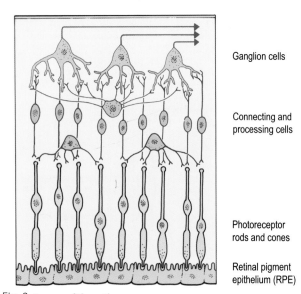

Fig. 2 **Layers of the retina.**

Drainage

Aqueous circulates from the posterior to the anterior chamber through the pupil, leaving the eye through the trabecular meshwork (Fig. 1). This is a specialised tissue in the anterior chamber angle between the iris and the cornea. It resembles a sieve. From here aqueous drains into Schlemm's canal, which rings the circumference of the eye at the corneoscleral limbus, subsequently draining into veins.

Aqueous production and drainage are balanced to maintain an appropriate intraocular pressure.

Vitreous

The vitreous body is 99% water but, vitally, also contains collagen fibrils and hyaluronan, which impart cohesion and a gel-like consistency. With increasing age, the vitreous undergoes progressive liquefaction (degeneration). The vitreous is adherent to the retina at certain points, particularly at the optic disc and at the ora serrata. When the vitreous degenerates, it can pull on the retina, cause a tear and lead to retinal detachment. The vitreous helps to cushion the eye during trauma and has a minor role as a metabolic sump.

Retina

The retina (Fig. 2) converts focused light images into nerve impulses. It comprises the neurosensory retina and the retinal pigment epithelium (RPE). Light has to pass through the inner retina to reach the photoreceptors, the rods and cones, which convert light energy into electrical energy (Table 1). The retina therefore has to be transparent. Connector neurones modify and pass on the electrical signals to the ganglion cells, whose axons run along the surface of the retina and enter the optic nerve.

An area called the macula provides for central vision. At its centre is a specialised area, the fovea, which is for high quality vision. The rest of the retina is for peripheral vision (Fig. 3).

Cones, concentrated at the macula, are responsible for fine vision (acuity) and colour appreciation. Rods are for vision in low light levels and the detection of movement. They are distributed throughout the entire retina. Photoreceptors contain visual pigments comprising retinol (vitamin A) linked to protein (opsin). Light absorption causes structural and then a chemical change in visual pigments which results in electrical hyperpolarisation of the photoreceptor.

External to the neurosensory retina lies the RPE, a single layer of pigmented cells which are essential to photoreceptor physiology. RPE cells recycle vitamin A for the formation of photopigments, transport water and metabolites, renew photoreceptors and help to reduce damage by scattered light. Impairment of RPE function, which can occur with age and in many disease states, can lead to loss of retinal function and, therefore, sight.

The blood supply of the retina is derived from the central retinal artery and vein, and from the choroid. Both systems are required for normal function. The retinal vessels enter and leave the eye through the optic nerve and run in the nerve fibre layer. A major arterial and venous branch, forming an 'arcade', supplies each of the retinal quadrants.

The blood–retinal barrier, consisting of tight junctions between the endothelial cells of the retinal vessels and between the RPE cells, isolates the retinal environment from the systemic circulation. Disruption of the barriers, as occurs in diabetic retinopathy, leads to retinal oedema and precipitation of lipid and protein, causing loss of retinal transparency and therefore loss of vision.

Optic nerve

The ganglion cell axons in the retinal nerve fibre layer make a right-angled turn into the optic nerve at the optic disc, which has no photoreceptor and corresponds to the physiological blind spot (Fig. 3). Most optic discs have a central cavity, the optic cup, which is pale in comparison with the redness of the surrounding nerve fibres. Loss of nerve fibres, as occurs in glaucoma, results in an increase in the volume of the cup.

There are about one million axons in the optic nerve. Behind the eyeball these axons become myelinated. Here the optic nerve is surrounded by cerebrospinal fluid in an anterior extension of the subarachnoid space and is protected by the same membranous layers as the brain.

Table 1 **Properties of rods and cones**		
	Rods	**Cones**
Function	Vision in dim light, movement high resolution	Vision in bright light, colour,
Total number	>100 million	6–7 million
Highest density	Peripheral retina	Macula

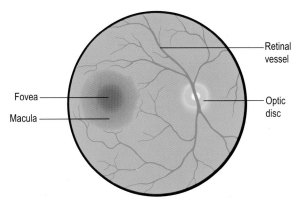

Fig. 3 **Diagram of the retina** (right eye).

Fovea — Macula — Retinal vessel — Optic disc

Anatomy and physiology: inner eye

- Iris: constriction is parasympathetic, dilation sympathetic.
- Ciliary body: forms aqueous humour; mediates accommodation (active–parasympathetic).
- Lens: consists of a hard nucleus and softer cortex, bounded by a capsule and held in place by the zonules.
- Aqueous drains through the trabecular meshwork in the anterior chamber angle between the iris and cornea.
- Retina:
  – Requires intact retinal and choroidal vasculature and retinal pigment epithelial layer for normal function.
  – Photoreceptors convert light energy into electrical; transmit to ganglion cells via connector neurones.
  – Ganglion cell axons pass across the surface of the retina and leave the eye at the optic disc.
  – Cone photoreceptors are concentrated at the macula for high quality colour vision.

Relations and connections: orbit and visual pathways

Each eye lies within a bony socket, the orbit, which protects the eyeball in all directions apart from the front. The muscles which move the eye attach within the orbit. Within the orbit are motor, sensory and autonomic nerves to the eyeball and associated structures. Space between these structures is filled with fat and a complex array of connective tissue fibres which help to suspend the eye above the floor of the orbit and interact with the extraocular muscles.

Our field and quality of vision is improved by having two eyes. The optic nerves from each eye are coordinated intracranially and connected with other areas of the cerebral cortex. The result is 'sight'. A set of motor centres, cranial nerve nuclei and connections harness the two eyes together, like the front wheels of a car, to maintain binocular vision without diplopia (binocular single vision).

The orbit

The bony walls of the orbit form a pyramidal structure. They are the frontal, maxillary, zygomatic, ethmoid, lacrimal and sphenoid bones (Fig. 1). The medial wall and the floor of the orbit are thin. When a forceful blow to the eye forces it back into the orbit, decompression through fracture of the floor or medial wall minimises damage to the eyeball. On the other hand, infection in the maxillary or ethmoid sinus can easily spread into the orbit.

At the apex of the orbit, the optic foramen conveys the optic nerve backwards to the intracranial optic chiasm, and the ophthalmic artery forward into the orbit. Lateral to the foramen are two fissures:

- The superior orbital fissure provides passage for the lacrimal, frontal and nasociliary nerves (ophthalmic division of the fifth cranial nerve), the third, fourth and sixth cranial nerves, and the superior ophthalmic vein passing to the cavernous sinus.
- The inferior orbital fissure permits exit of the inferior ophthalmic vein from the orbit and entry of the maxillary division of the fifth cranial nerve (thus a fracture of the floor of the orbit can cause abnormal sensation on the cheek).

The four extraocular rectus muscles form a cone within which are the sensory and autonomic nerves and arteries to the eyeball, including the optic nerve and the motor nerves to all the extraocular muscles including the levator but excluding the superior oblique. Thus, compression at the

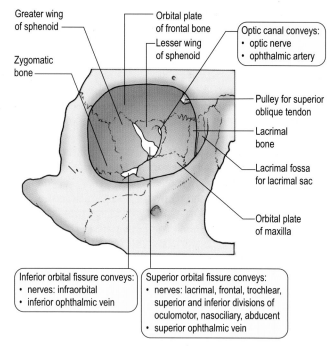

Fig. 1 **The right bony orbit.**

Labels:
Greater wing of sphenoid
Zygomatic bone
Orbital plate of frontal bone
Lesser wing of sphenoid
Optic canal conveys:
- optic nerve
- ophthalmic artery
Pulley for superior oblique tendon
Lacrimal bone
Lacrimal fossa for lacrimal sac
Orbital plate of maxilla

Inferior orbital fissure conveys:
- nerves: infraorbital
- inferior ophthalmic vein

Superior orbital fissure conveys:
- nerves: lacrimal, frontal, trochlear, superior and inferior divisions of oculomotor, nasociliary, abducent
- superior ophthalmic vein

orbital apex, for example by a tumour, may result in loss of corneal sensation, reduced ocular movement and impaired visual function, as well as displacement of the globe forwards (proptosis). Complete ocular anaesthesia by injection requires that the local anaesthetic be placed or diffused into this intraconal space.

Extraocular muscles

The four rectus muscles have a common posterior attachment to a ring of connective tissue which surrounds the optic foramen. They pass forwards around the eyeball to insert 5–7 mm behind the limbus (Fig. 2). Their features are listed in Table 1.

Levator muscle

Levator muscle (third nerve) passes forward and widens into a broad aponeurosis, attaching to the superior tarsal plate and eyelid skin. There are some associated smooth muscle fibres innervated by the sympathetic nervous system.

Table 1 **The extraocular muscles**				
Muscle	Origin	Insertion	Nerve supply	Action
Medial rectus	Orbital apex	Medial to corneoscleral junction (limbus)	Third cranial (oculomotor) nerve	Moves the eye medially (adduction)
Lateral rectus	Orbital apex	Lateral to limbus	Sixth cranial (abducens) nerve	Moves the eye laterally (abduction)
Superior rectus	Orbital apex	Superior to limbus	Oculomotor nerve	*Main:* elevation *Additional:* adduction, intorsion (inward rotation)
Inferior rectus	Orbital apex	Inferior to limbus	Oculomotor nerve	*Main:* depression *Additional:* adduction, extorsion (outward rotation)
Superior oblique	Medial to orbital apex, passing through a pulley (trochlea) attached behind superonasal orbital rim	Travels backwards from trochlea to attach superiorly behind the equator of the eyeball	Fourth cranial (trochlear) nerve	*Main:* intorsion *Additional:* abduction, depression
Inferior oblique	Behind inferonasal orbital rim	Inferiorly behind the equator	Oculomotor nerve	*Main:* extorsion *Additional:* abduction, elevation

Nerves of the orbit

In addition to the motor nerves to the extraocular muscles the orbit contains sensory and autonomic nerves (Fig. 2).

The chief sensory nerve is of course the optic nerve. It is enclosed within a sheath continuous with the intracranial meninges, so that the subarachnoid space extends right up to the globe. Its blood supply comes from numerous vessels derived from the ophthalmic artery. At its anterior end, this blood supply is not anastomotic, so that disruption by an ischaemic process such as atherosclerosis or giant cell arteritis typically causes severe visual loss.

Branches of the ophthalmic division of the trigeminal (fifth) nerve are sensory to the eyeball (especially the cornea), the conjunctiva and the skin of the eyelids extending up across the forehead and back towards the occiput. Hence, varicella-zoster virus infection (shingles) of this division causes a widespread dermatomal rash. The nasociliary nerve is the branch to the eyeball, but it does not terminate there. The nerve passes on into the medial orbital wall and emerges on the side of the nose. Shingles affecting the eyeball usually causes a rash in this area of skin also.

The parasympathetic nerve fibres to the ciliary body (accommodation) and iris constrictor muscles travel with the third nerve. There is a synapse between pre- and postganglionic fibres in the ciliary ganglion close to the optic nerve.

Parasympathetic fibres to the lacrimal gland pursue a complex course, passing with the facial nerve and then following the maxillary division of the trigeminal.

The sensory and parasympathetic nerve fibres reach the eyeball via the short and long ciliary nerves which pierce the sclera posteriorly.

Post-ganglionic sympathetic fibres arise in the superior cervical ganglion in the neck, latch on to the internal carotid artery and run a long course, entering the cranium, passing through the cavernous sinus and entering the orbit. In addition to being vasoconstrictor to arteries, they innervate the ciliary body (production of aqueous humour) and the iris dilator muscle. Maximal pupil dilation can be achieved by the topical administration of an inhibitor of the parasympathetic system (such as the anticholinergics tropicamide and cyclopentolate) plus a sympathetic agonist (such as phenylephrine).

The visual pathways (see also p. 8)

The two optic nerves unite at the optic chiasm above the sella turcica of the

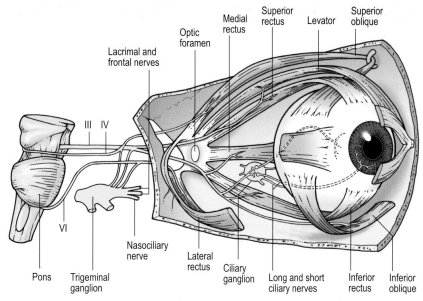

Fig. 2 **The nerves and muscles of the right orbit.**

sphenoid bone. The pituitary gland projects down immediately behind the chiasm. Nerve fibres from the nasal retina (temporal or lateral field of vision) cross over to the opposite side in the chiasm, so that the post-chiasmal fibres on the left subserve the field of vision on the right (and vice versa).

The optic tracts extend from the chiasm to the lateral geniculate body. Here, nerves which began as fibres on the surface of the retina form synapses with neurones passing through the optic radiation to reach the visual cortex in the occipital lobes.

Pressure on the chiasm by a pituitary tumour causes a bitemporal hemianopia. Behind the chiasm, a unilateral lesion causes a hemianopia on the opposite side.

There is topographic localisation of nerve fibres for areas of the visual field throughout the visual pathways, rather than a disorganised random mixing of nerve fibres. This means that focal damage causes a focal defect in the field of vision, the extent determined by the number of fibres damaged.

The optic tracts and radiations are supplied by branches of the middle cerebral artery, the visual cortex by the posterior cerebral artery. Each macula is represented by an extensive area of cortex at both occipital poles, which have a dual blood supply (the middle and posterior cerebral arteries). As a result, occlusion of the arterial supply to the visual cortex causes bilateral field loss which spares central vision (macular sparing).

Relation and connections: orbit and visual pathways

- The bony walls of the orbit are thin inferiorly and medially.
- The superior orbital fissure transmits the sensory nerves to the eye and orbit and the 3rd, 4th and 6th cranial nerves.
- The optic nerve and the ophthalmic artery pass through the optic foramen.
- The 3rd nerve supplies levator; superior, inferior and medial rectus; inferior oblique; accommodation; pupil constriction.
- The 4th nerve supplies superior oblique.
- The 6th nerve supplies lateral rectus.
- Extraocular muscle function: depends on the direction of gaze:
  - medial rectus: horizontal towards the nose
  - lateral rectus: horizontal laterally
  - obliques primarily rotate the eye
  - vertical recti primarily elevate/depress the eye.
- Visual pathways
  - optic nerve to chiasm (fibres from nasal retina cross over) to optic tract
  - synapse in lateral geniculate body
  - optic radiation to occipital cortex.

Human sight

Sight

The process leading to the perception of an image by the brain, 'sight', is extremely complex. It starts in the retina with the conversion of photons into electricity. This is achieved by light-sensitive visual pigments which contain retinal (the aldehyde of retinol, from vitamin A) and opsin (a protein). Light absorption results in a structural change in retinal, followed by a chemical change in the opsin. Ion channels in the photoreceptor cell membrane are altered and the cell becomes hyperpolarised. Rod photoreceptors contain rhodopsin which is stimulated by light of wavelength 505 nm. This is the wavelength at which the eye is maximally sensitive in dim light. There are three subsets of cone photoreceptor: each contains a pigment which is maximally sensitive to blue, green or red light. This is the basis for colour vision.

Adaptation to ambient light is an important physiological process. Dark adaptation takes several minutes, requiring regeneration of visual pigments, especially in rods.

There is some rudimentary image processing in the retina, based on colour, movement and position, which is achieved by having two types of photoreceptor, by the concentration of cones at the macula and by specialised connector neurones within the retina.

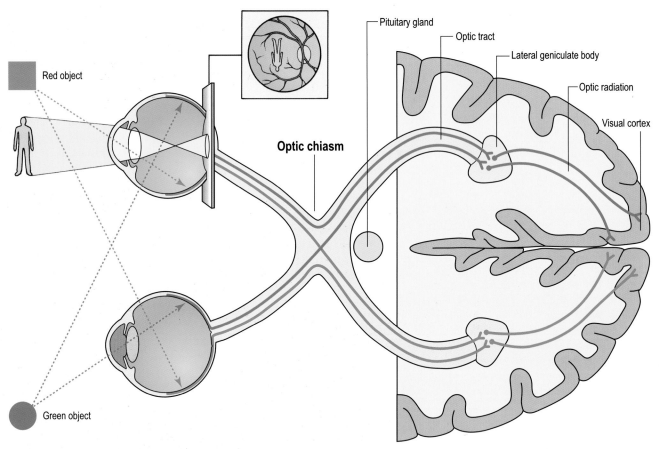

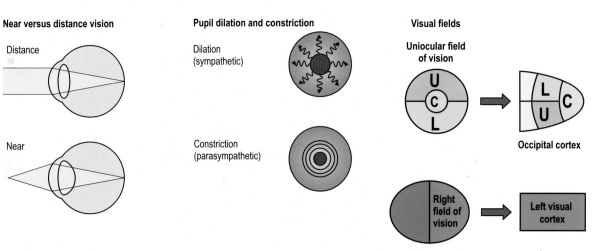

L = lower   C = central   U = upper

Further image processing occurs in the brain, at the lateral geniculate nucleus and in the visual cortex. The parietal lobes are important for recognition, orientation and motor tasks such as reading, writing and copying.

Throughout the course of the visual pathways, topographic representation of an image is maintained, so that a destructive lesion will result in a characteristic visual field defect.

Visual acuity

Visual acuity is a measure of the ability of the eye to see that two closely positioned objects are separate. The angle subtended at the normal eye by these two objects is on average 1 minute of arc. Letters on the Snellen chart are constructed as multiples of this angle at the standard test distance of 6 metres. Other tests of visual resolution exist: for example, contrast sensitivity which consists of a series of black lines of graduated contrast and separation.

Three-dimensional vision

Quality 3-D vision (stereopsis) occurs because the eyes are separated, so that each eye views the same object from a slightly different perspective. Both eyes must have good vision. However, depth perception does not depend entirely on the presence of two eyes. Monocular visual clues such as proximity, shadows, perspective, overlap and parallax assist in the interpretation of an object. Nevertheless, it can take a long time to adapt to the sudden loss of the sight of one eye.

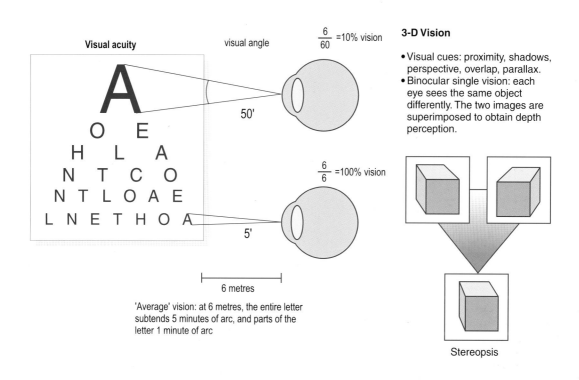

'Average' vision: at 6 metres, the entire letter subtends 5 minutes of arc, and parts of the letter 1 minute of arc

3-D Vision

- Visual cues: proximity, shadows, perspective, overlap, parallax.
- Binocular single vision: each eye sees the same object differently. The two images are superimposed to obtain depth perception.

Stereopsis

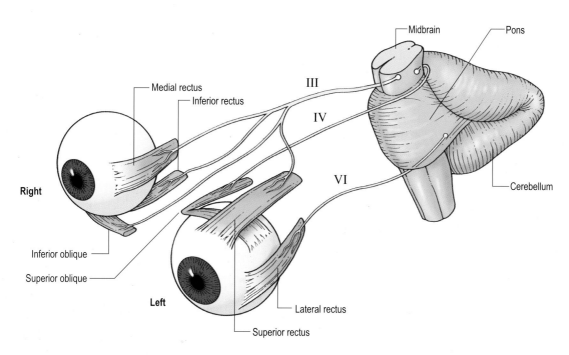

The ophthalmic history I

As in all areas of medicine, a careful history is of great importance in that it:

- may suggest the disease and its cause
- may identify parts of the clinical examination which need special attention
- may indicate a need for particular additional investigations
- should place the clinical ophthalmic problem in the context of the person as a whole
- may indicate conditions that can be modified for prevention of future diseases (ocular as well as non-ocular).

History of the complaint

The broad spectrum of ocular disease usually presents as a combination of a relatively small number of symptoms.

Typically, this might be a change in vision or reddening of one or both eyes. Sometimes the patient is asymptomatic, an optometrist or other professional having detected an abnormality on routine examination.

Specific points to be considered in the history of each of the main clinical problems are detailed in Figures 1–9. These can be used as a guide to approaching the scenarios presented in the Clinical Decision-Making section at the end of this book.

It is important to determine the functional impact of the condition. This is particularly important in the elderly person with cataract. Many elderly people have cataract but removal may not always be necessary. Ask about indicators of function, such as reading, crossing the road and shopping.

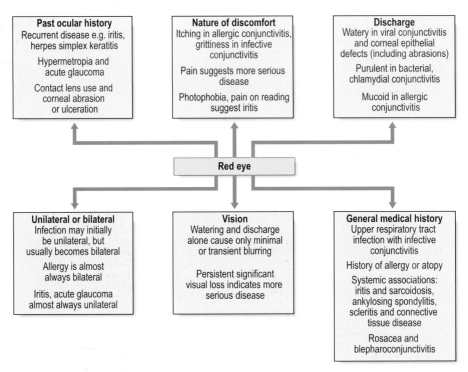

Fig. 1 **Red eye.**

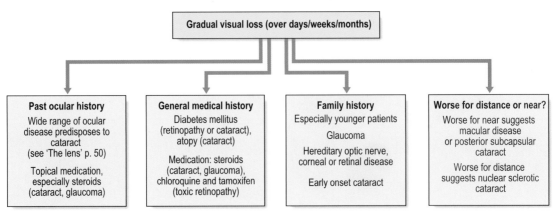

Fig. 2 **Gradual visual loss.**

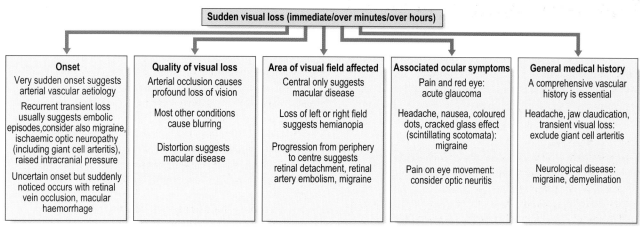

Fig. 3 **Sudden visual loss.**

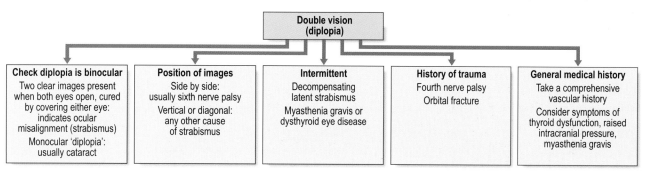

Fig. 4 **Diplopia.**

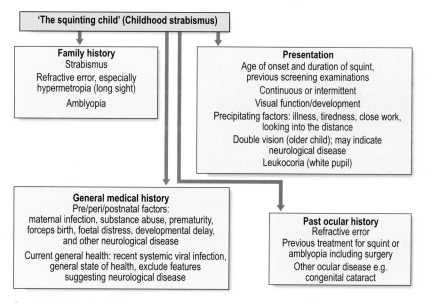

Fig. 5 **Childhood strabismus.**

The ophthalmic history II

Past ocular history

In cases of gradual visual loss, you should ensure that the patient has had a recent sight test (refraction) in order to exclude an uncorrected refractive error. The refractive state of the eye may be associated with certain pathologies:

- myopia with retinal detachment and early-onset vitreous degeneration causing floaters
- hypermetropia with acute angle closure glaucoma and pseudopapilloedema.

A history of amblyopia (lazy eye) should be elicited, not least because the person presenting with symptoms in the fellow non-amblyopic eye will be especially anxious. With this in mind it is useful in visual loss to be certain of the childhood quality of vision in each eye. Some conditions are recurrent, such as iritis and herpes simplex keratitis. Trauma can lead to cataract, glaucoma and retinal detachment.

Family history

Some rare conditions have a simple pattern of inheritance, but others have a less well-defined familial association, such as presenile cataract and primary open angle glaucoma, the incidence of which is higher than average in close family members.

General history

This may be brief or exhaustive, depending on the reason for the patient assessment. A range of ophthalmic conditions are manifestations of, or are associated with systemic disease. A vascular history is often mandatory: diabetes, hypertension, ischaemic heart disease, smoking, peripheral vascular disease, plasma lipid status, cerebrovascular disease, etc. Ask about heart and lung disease: topical beta-blockers for glaucoma should not be prescribed to the patient with asthma and only with caution in those with heart problems. The patient due to have surgery requires a history that addresses potential general or local anaesthetic problems.

Allergy and current medication

Many topically applied drugs and their delivery vehicles and preservatives may stimulate an allergic reaction which should be considered in the patient with a persistent red eye.

Interactions between systemically administered medications and topical ophthalmic preparations are very rare, but systemic drugs are sometimes used to treat ophthalmic disease.

A drug history may reveal the patient who has reversible airways disease but denies a history of asthma!

Social history

Smoking and alcohol consumption are associated with many diseases, and ophthalmic disease is no exception.

Knowledge of the patient's social situation is especially important when considering arrangements for surgery (such as their suitability for day case surgery) and in assessing and counselling the patient with severe irreversible visual loss.

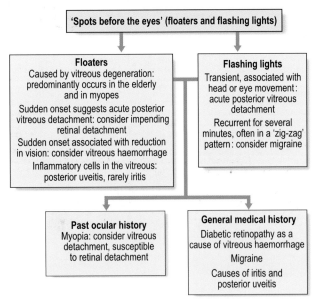

Fig. 6 **Floaters and flashing lights.**

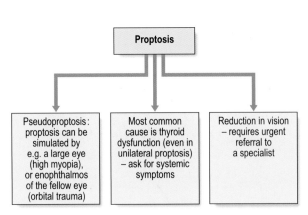

Fig. 7 **Proptosis.**

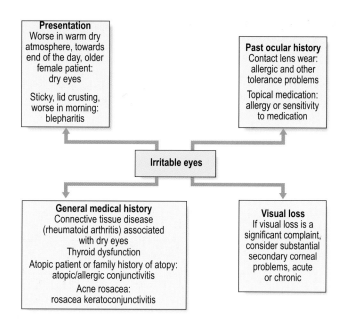

Fig. 8 **Irritable eyes.**

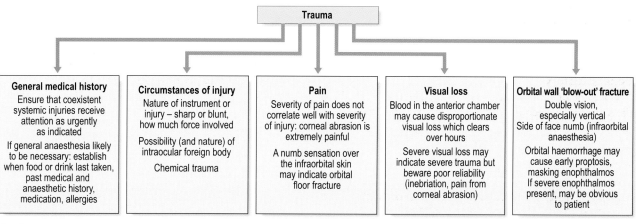

Fig. 9 **Trauma.**

The ophthalmic history

- Red eye without discharge may suggest serious disease.

- Visual loss
  - in red eye, indicates serious ocular disease
  - differentiate between sudden and gradual.

- Eye pain
  - differentiate between discomfort/irritation and deep pain
  - true pain suggests serious disease.

- The services of an interpreter may be necessary to obtain a good history in the presence of a language barrier.

The ophthalmic examination

Once an appropriate history has been taken, a simple examination should lead to a short list of diagnostic possibilities. It is helpful to consider that there is a 'basic' examination, which all practitioners can complete, and a 'specialist' examination, usually performed by an ophthalmologist.

The basic examination

Equipment

- chart and pinhole aperture for measuring visual acuity
- light, such as a pen torch
- target such as a hat pin for testing the visual field
- occluder for cover testing
- fluorescein and dilating drops
- direct ophthalmoscope.

Testing vision

There are three elements of vision: acuity, field and colour.

Visual acuity

This is tested using a Snellen chart comprising lines of high contrast letters decreasing in size from the top to the bottom of the chart. Each line is labelled with the distance in metres at which it should be seen by the normally sighted eye. For the test to be reliable, the chart should be illuminated from behind and the subject should be at a specified distance, usually 3 or 6 metres. First test acuity with spectacles, if available, then with a pinhole. The pinhole vision suggests the best visual acuity which might be achieved with correct spectacle lenses. The acuity is recorded as a fraction: the subject's distance from the chart as the numerator and the line seen as the denominator. For example, the 9 metre line read at 6 metres is recorded as 6/9. 'Normal' visual acuity is age-dependent:

- 6/4–6/6 for a young person
- 6/9–6/12 for an elderly person.

Table 1 **The basic examination**

- Visual acuity and visual fields
- Double vision: cover test and eye movements
- The outer eye
  - for redness and discharge
  - for corneal clarity/ulceration
- The inner eye
  - pupil responses, shape, symmetry
  - red reflex
  - optic disc, macula; peripheral retina

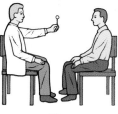

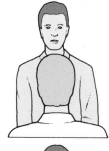

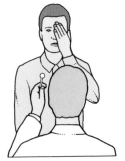

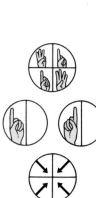

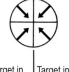

Target in L hand | Target in R hand

Fig. 1 **Visual field testing.**

Principles
Sit at same level, faces 1m apart.
Subject covers his eye with own hand of same side.
Compare your field with the subject's field :
-his R with your L
-his L with your R
Move target slowly, equidistant between the two of you

Steps
1. Both eyes open
'Look at my nose. Is any part of my face missing?'
Detects central scotoma, hemianopia

2. Each eye in turn
a) Finger counting in quadrants
'How many fingers do you see?'
Detects hemianopias, quadrantanopias
b) Compare R and L hemifields simultaneously with one finger
'Which finger is most clear?'
Detects less dense hemianopia
3. Each eye in turn
Bring target in from periphery
'Point when you first see the target'
Detects quadrantanopias, altitudinal defects, even paracentral scotomas

Visual field

Large dense defects of the visual field are easily identified using a simple confrontational technique (Fig. 1). More subtle defects can also be demonstrated with care, patience and attention to detail.

Colour

Asymmetry of colour appreciation can be tested using a bright red target. A more objective test requires an aid such as the Ishihara colour plates.

Ocular motility

A complaint of double vision in an adult or a suspicion of 'squint' (strabismus) in a child means that an assessment of the position and movement of the two eyes in relation to each other is necessary. The first step is to look for asymmetry of the corneal light reflex with a pen torch. A cover test should then be performed, followed by observation of the movement of the eyes as they move into the key positions of gaze (Fig. 2).

The outer eye

A pen torch or direct ophthalmoscope provides adequate illumination. The examination should follow an anatomical sequence – eyelids, conjunctiva, cornea. Key signs to detect are:

- presence and distribution of any inflammation
- discharge
- loss of corneal clarity
- corneal ulceration.

Fluorescein drops are a useful diagnostic aid. Fluorescein mixes into the tear film and adheres to areas of epithelial loss (ulcer or abrasion). It is best visualised using a blue light. Your pen torch should have a blue filter, and many ophthalmoscopes now incorporate one.

The inner eye

Again, it is wise to apply a logical sequence to the examination. The direct ophthalmoscope is required. Test the pupils, look at the red reflex and then examine the fundus (retina and optic disc).

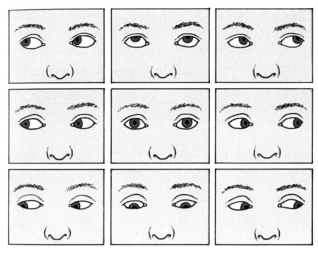

Fig. 2 **Testing of ocular movement.**

The normal pupil constricts in response to light (the direct reflex). The pupil of the fellow eye will also constrict (the consensual reflex). A useful but difficult test to perform is the swinging flashlight test for a relative afferent pupil defect (RAPD), which usually indicates unilateral optic nerve pathology (though extensive retinal disease will also cause a positive response).

The more frequent abnormalities you will encounter are asymmetry of pupil size, reduced reactivity and irregularity of shape.

The red reflex is seen when light enters the pupil and is reflected from the retina. It is commonly seen in flash photography by compact cameras. Anything which interferes with the passage of light will diminish the red reflex, but the main cause is cataract.

Examination of the ocular fundus (back of the eye – the retina and optic disc) is greatly simplified by attention to a few simple rules:

- dilate the pupils with drops
- reduce random eye movement: ensure that the patient's other eye fixes on an object which is located straight ahead and a little higher than the line of sight

Table 2 **Interpretation of findings**

Findings	Interpretation
Visual acuity less than expected	
Does it improve with pinhole?	Suggests new spectacles required
Is there a normal red reflex?	No, consider cataract
	Yes, consider retinal or optic nerve disease
Abnormal visual fields	
Monocular	Optic nerve or retinal pathology
Binocular	Intracranial disease
Inflammation	
Entire conjunctiva (globe and lid)	Conjunctivitis (infective, allergic)
Confined to the eyeball	Check the cornea
	Consider iritis, episcleritis, acute glaucoma
Corneal fluorescein staining	Indicates abrasion/ulceration
	Look for infiltration, suggesting infection
Pupil asymmetry	
Direct and consensual reactions normal?	Yes, likely to be non-pathological asymmetry
Larger pupil fails to constrict	Efferent pathway disorder — exclude oculomotor nerve palsy
Small and/or irregular	Iritis, prior surgery
Diminished red reflex	Usually lens opacity (cataract)
	Corneal opacity obscures the iris and pupil
	Vitreous opacities swirl as the eye moves
Retinal pathology	Define the location of the abnormality
	Describe the appearance — pigmentation, atrophy, haemorrhage, exudate
	Is it bilateral?

- find the optic disc; follow the vessels away from the disc and then back again; track horizontally and laterally from the disc to locate the macula.

Non-ophthalmologists fear to dilate pupils because of the overstated risk of preciptating acute angle closure glaucoma. In fact, the risk of failure to identify retinal or optic nerve disease by not dilating the pupils is considerably greater than that of inducing glaucoma.

Systemic examination

Many ocular conditions are associated with systemic disease. The need for a systemic examination will therefore be determined by the ocular clinical findings.

Specialist techniques

The slit lamp

The slit lamp (Fig. 3), a horizontally mounted binocular microscope, is the most important of the instruments used to examine the eye in more detail. It is so called because the illuminating beam can be reduced to a vertical slit. Directed at the eye at an angle of approximately 45 degrees from the observer's eyepieces, an optical sagittal section of the eye is achieved.

The slit lamp provides a highly magnified and stereoscopic view. The basic apparatus enables only the anterior part of the eye, as far back as the lens, to be focused. A variety of supplementary lenses, both contact and non-contact, can be used to examine the entire inner eye.

Non-specialist use of the slit lamp is useful in the general accident and emergency department, for examination of the cornea and for localisation and removal of foreign bodies.

Tonometry

Tonometry (measurement of the intraocular pressure) can be performed with a device attached to the slit lamp or with a handheld electronic gauge. Both require contact with the cornea and, therefore, topical anaesthesia. High street optometrists generally use a non-contact air-puff tonometer.

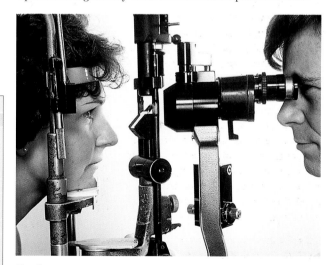

Fig. 3 **Use of the slit lamp.**

> ### The ophthalmic examination
>
> - A simple clinical examination includes:
>   - measurement of visual function (acuity, fields to confrontation, colour, pupil reactions)
>   - assessment of eye position and movement
>   - examination of the outer eye, looking for inflammation, discharge, fluorescein staining of the cornea, corneal clarity
>   - pupil dilation, followed by assessment of the clarity of the ocular media and examination of the retina.
>
> - The slit lamp is used for binocular magnified examination of the eye, including the entire interior.

Special investigations

A variety of investigative techniques are available to help with assessment and management and to improve quantitative recording.

Amsler grid

This is a 10 cm x 10 cm line grid comprising 0.5 cm squares (Fig. 1). The subject holds the chart at a comfortable reading distance with one eye covered, and fixes on the dot at the centre of the grid. The grid area corresponds roughly with that of the macula. Any significant macular disease will usually be apparent as a distortion or as a missing area (scotoma).

Tests for colour vision

A simple clinical test is to compare the hue of a red pen top between each eye. Pseudoisochromatic plates such as the Ishihara series (Fig. 2), which were developed to test for inherited defects of colour vision, can be used to identify acquired defects. More accurate and specific colour vision tests are available, such as the Farnsworth-Munsell 100 Hue Test.

Exophthalmometer

The exophthalmometer (Fig. 3) measures the position of the anterior surface of the corneas relative to the lateral orbital rims in the assessment of proptosis.

Refraction

Refraction refers to the determination of the refractive error of the eyes, principally to facilitate spectacle or contact lens prescription. It is most commonly performed as part of the 'eye test' carried out by optometrists (ophthalmic opticians). The refractive error can be estimated by a machine, an autorefractor, although confirmation and refinement by a practitioner is required. Refraction is essential in determining the best corrected visual acuity, especially when the vision improves with a pinhole.

Assessment of corneal power and shape

Evaluation of corneal disease and planning of surgery to the anterior segment, including refractive surgery, requires measurement of corneal curvature and power (keratometry). This can be achieved by the projection of illuminated shapes (mires) onto the cornea, such as Placido's disc of concentric black and white circles. Computerised systems are now available which enhance the detailed analysis of shape and refractive power (Fig. 4).

Biometry

This is the process by which the required dioptric power of an

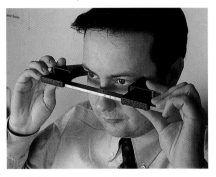

Fig. 3 **Use of an exophthalmometer.**

intraocular lens implant is calculated prior to cataract surgery. Biometry involves estimation of corneal power and measurement of the axial length of the eye using an ultrasonic scanner, an A-scan.

Orthoptics

An orthoptist is concerned with the non-medical aspects of the assessment, monitoring and treatment of ocular motility and related disorders, particularly childhood concomitant strabismus and amblyopia.

Techniques and equipment used by orthoptists include prismatic measurement of ocular deviation, the Hess chart (a graphical representation of eye movement) and tests of 3-dimensional vision.

Perimetry

Formal plotting of the visual fields, or perimetry, is most frequently performed as part of a glaucoma assessment. Perimeters, which may be manually operated or automated, present either

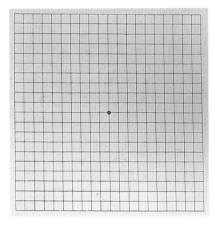

Fig. 1 **Amsler chart.**

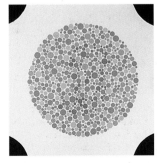

Fig. 2 **Ishihara pseudoisochromatic plates.**

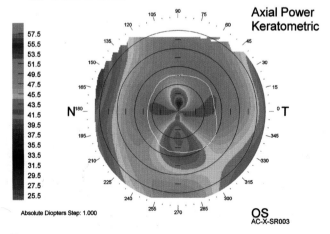

Fig. 4 **Corneal contour chart produced by computed tomography.**

static or kinetic stimuli. Kinetic stimuli are moved into a 'seeing' area from a 'non-seeing' area. In static perimetry, the stimulus brightness at, typically, 40 locations is changed until it is detected by the subject. An automated field analyser also monitors subject reliability and statistically analyses data.

Fundus fluorescein angiography (FFA)
The passage of fluorescent dye, injected into a peripheral vein, through the blood vessels of the fundus can be recorded by a still or video camera. In the normal eye, fluorescein will remain within the retinal blood vessels (Fig. 5). Many fundus abnormalities can be defined as areas of hypo- or hyper-fluorescence. For instance, retinal ischaemia will show as hypofluorescence, and diabetic microaneurysms which leak dye are hyperfluorescent. FFA is especially useful in the assessment of 'wet' age-related macular degeneration, which may be treatable by laser photocoagulation.

Indocyanine green (ICG) fundus angiography provides information about the choroidal circulation and may be used as an adjunct to FFA.

Electrophysiological testing
Electrophysiological tests provide an objective evaluation of the function of the visual pathways by measuring electrical responses to light stimuli. Several are in common clinical use. Visual evoked response (VER) testing gauges the function of the optic nerve and the macula by detecting changes in visual cortex electrical potential to visual stimuli. A typical use of the VER is to confirm a previous episode of optic neuritis. Electroretinography (ERG) and electro-oculography (EOG) are used to evaluate the neuroretina and the retinal

pigment epithelium respectively, generally in the context of inherited retinal disease such as retinitis pigmentosa. Multifocal ERG tests individual retinal locations and may in the future allow objective visual field assessment.

Ultrasonic imaging
The 'A-scan' ocular ultrasound facility provides a one-dimensional graphical representation of the ocular media. Its main use is the measurement of the axial length of the eye to aid the calculation of the power of an intraocular lens for implantation.

The 'B-scan' facility provides a two-dimensional image (Fig. 6). It is especially useful when an opacity, commonly vitreous haemorrhage or dense cataract, prevents optical visualisation of the fundus to exclude posterior segment pathology such as a retinal detachment. The B-scan can also be used tao provide limited information about pathology of the optic nerve and orbit. Ultrasound biomicroscopy (UBM) is a high resolution scanner of anterior ocular structures such as the anterior chamber angle and ciliary body.

CT and MR imaging
The orbit, including the optic nerve and the extraocular muscles, is best imaged by computed tomographic (CT) and magnetic resonance (MR) techniques. CT is particularly suitable for assessment of the bony orbit, whereas MRI is probably more useful than CT for acquiring information about the orbital soft tissues. Both modalities are invaluable for imaging the central nervous system.

Plain X-rays have largely been superseded in ophthalmology by other imaging methods but retain limited applicability in some circumstances,

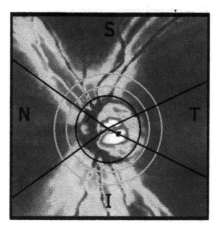
Fig. 7 **Scanning laser polarimetry of left eye retina.** Nerve layer thickness is colour-coded.

notably in trauma assessment where they may be used to screen for major bony damage or for radio-opaque foreign bodies.

Imaging the optic nerve and retina
Optical coherence tomography (OCT), scanning laser ophthalmoscopy (SLO) and scanning laser polarimetry (SLP) (Fig. 7) are new techniques for precise measurement of retinal thickness and optic disc neuroretinal rim area and volume. They may differentiate normal from abnormal appearances and detect change in structure with time, for example, in the management of glaucoma.

Lacrimal drainage imaging
Clinical examination is usually sufficient to guide the management of lacrimal drainage obstruction, but in some cases it is helpful to supplement this by means of dacryocystography, using X-rays and a contrast medium, or scintillography in which tears are labelled with a radio-isotope. Endoscopic visualisation of the lacrimal system is now possible.

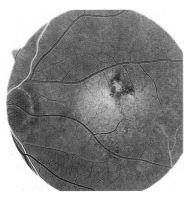
Fig. 5 **Fundus fluorescein angiogram.** The dye (black) has filled the arteries but not the veins. There is an abnormality at the macula.

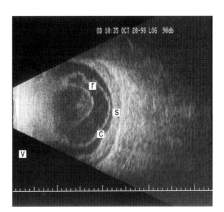
Fig. 6 **'B-scan' ultrasonic image of a normal eye.** V: vitreous cortex; c: choroid; s: sclera; r: retina.

Special investigations
- Special ophthalmic investigations are frequently necessary to supplement clinical information.
- Range from simple tests requiring a minimum of apparatus to advanced technology.
- An important example is fundus fluorescein angiography, which forms an integral part of the management of many retinal conditions.

Ocular pathology

This spread describes some of the many aspects of pathology particular to the eye and its surrounding structures, together with the histopathology of certain important diseases.

Repair and destruction: the diseased eye

Ocular inflammation

Physiological barriers isolate the eye from the systemic circulation: the blood–aqueous barrier, and the inner and outer blood–retinal barriers. The blood–aqueous barrier comprises 'tight' junctions between cells of the ciliary body and tight junctions between endothelial cells of iris blood vessels. The inner blood–retinal barrier consists of tight junctions between retinal vascular endothelial cells; the outer barrier is made by tight junctions between retinal pigment epithelial cells, preventing diffusion from the choroid. Together, these barriers help to control the composition of the intraocular fluids, preventing escape of proteins and cells from the circulation. The barriers are breached in inflammation, destabilising this carefully controlled environment and exacerbating the primary inflammatory stimulus.

This concept of a carefully maintained intraocular environment in which reparative processes may result in tissue disruption is crucial to an understanding of the functional consequences and management of ocular disease. In most parts of the body, inflammation is a necessary route to recovery, but in the eye it can lead to cataract, glaucoma, macular oedema, retinal detachment and corneal scarring, amongst others, hence the very common use in ophthalmology of topical steroids to suppress inflammation.

Abnormal vascularisation

The vascular supply to the eye is carefully organised to maintain the chief function of the eye, vision. The cornea, lens and vitreous are avascular, and the retinal vessels are so positioned that they do not interfere with image formation by the transparent retina. A number of processes may result in abnormal vascularisation of the eye, including inflammation and ischaemia. In the cornea, vessels leak lipid and cause opacity; at the vitreoretinal interface they bleed (vitreous haemorrhage) or contract, detaching the retina.

Retinal disease

The retinal pigment epithelium (RPE) is a specialised cellular monolayer between the neurosensory retina and the choroid. It has many functions, including phagocytosis of debris and maintenance of the normal physiology of the rods and cones. In disease of the choroid and retina, the RPE cells replicate and migrate. The ophthalmoscopic signs of such processes are atrophy (loss of pigmentation) and hyperpigmentation.

Age-related macular degeneration, almost a 'normal' part of ageing, is a disorder in which the RPE is unable to maintain the normal function of the macular rods and cones. Loss of central vision is the result.

Corneal infection

The consequences of corneal infection are a good example of successful repair which results in functional failure. The response to the presence of microorganisms is inflammation: the transparent cornea is opacified by invasion of inflammatory cells. As the microorganisms are successfully cleared, fibroblast-like cells (keratocytes) lay down and re-model extracellular matrix, which is disorganised and therefore not transparent. Blood vessels grow in, contributing to the increase in cellularity, and leak protein and lipid. The

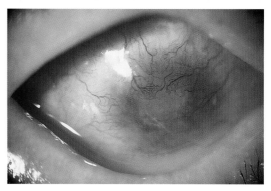

Fig. 1 **A vascularised corneal scar.**

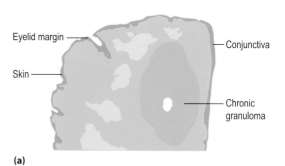

(a)

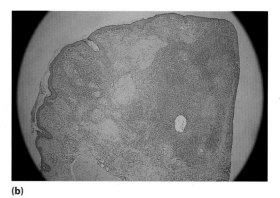

(b)

Fig. 2 **A chalazion.**

end result is scarring and loss of vision (Fig. 1). The normal cornea is an immunologically privileged site which tolerates the presence of foreign antigen. However, the presence of blood vessels reduces this tolerance, so that if corneal transplantation is performed to remove the scar, the risk of allograft rejection is greatly increased.

Systemic disease and immune processes

Many abnormalities of the eye are manifestations of systemic disease. In diabetic retinopathy, the pathological consequences of microangiopathy, namely vessel incompetence (leakage) and occlusion (ischaemia), lead directly to the physical signs seen on ophthalmoscopy. The same is true of hypertension. The angiopathic consequences of atherosclerosis may lead to loss of neural function: ischaemic optic neuropathy (blindness), visual pathway 'stroke' (field defect) and extraocular muscle nerve palsy (double vision).

Systemic inflammatory diseases, which are often autoimmune, may manifest in the eye. The primary site for this inflammation is frequently the uvea (the choroids, ciliary body and iris). Anteriorly, the most common site of involvement, inflammation gives the clinical syndrome of 'iritis' with protein exudation and cellular invasion into the anterior chamber. Posteriorly, choroidal inflammation disrupts normal retinal function. Retinal vasculitis and corneoscleral destruction may also occur.

Allergy

Allergy (hypersensitivity) is an excessive or altered reaction to antigen. Four types (I, II, III, IV) are recognised, all of which can affect the eye (typically the anterior segment), and there is often overlap between types. Allergic reactions may be acute (short-lived) or chronic. Whatever the duration, long-term sequelae can occur through damage to delicate conjunctival and corneal structures.

Hay fever is an example of a type I reaction. It is short-lived and resolves without significant structural damage. Atopic keratoconjunctivitis is a mixture of type I and IV processes, and frequently leads to corneal and conjunctival disruption and scarring.

Histopathology

Eyelids

Blockage of a meibomian gland may result in a chronic inflammatory nodule called a chalazion (Fig. 2). It consists of chronic granulomatous inflammation surrounding fat-filled spaces.

Xanthelasmata are dermal collections of lipid which may be associated with hyperlipidaemia.

The orbit

Dermoid cysts (page 33) result from imperfect fusion of embryonal skin flaps. They are lined by squamous epithelium and are filled with keratin. A dermoid may extend backwards deep into the orbit.

Swelling of the lacrimal gland may be inflammatory or may be due to a benign or malignant tumour. Benign pleomorphic adenoma of the lacrimal gland may recur if not completely removed at operation. Malignant lacrimal tumours (adenocarcinoma) cause pain and spread into adjacent bone.

Within the orbit, any structure may give rise to a benign or malignant space-occupying lesion. Of particular interest are varices (enlargements of pre-existing venous channels), cavernous haemangioma, rhabdomyosarcoma and pseudotumour. Cavernous haemangioma is the most common benign orbital tumour in adulthood. Rhabdomyosarcoma is a rare aggressive malignant tumour of an extraocular muscle occurring in childhood. It may mimic orbital cellulitis. So-called pseudotumour comprises a variety of processes, including lymphocytic infiltration, myositis and progressive fibrosis. Biopsy may show no abnormality at all.

The eyeball

Melanoma (Fig. 3) and retinoblastoma are the main primary tumours occurring within the eye. There are several histological types of choroidal melanoma (Fig. 4): some cell types are more aggressive than others. Melanoma may spread locally and to distant sites. Retinoblastoma (Fig. 5) is a malignant tumour of the retina, its cells characteristically grouping into clusters known as rosettes. Most occur sporadically in childhood but some are inherited as autosomal dominant defects, in which case they are often bilateral. There is a high incidence of second primary tumours in other sites.

Lymphoproliferative disease

Lymphoproliferative infiltrations may occur within the eye and mimic a uveitis. They may also occur in the conjunctiva and within the orbit, diffusely or in the lacrimal gland. On histological examination some are frankly malignant. Others appear to be reactive inflammation but later present as systemic lymphoma. Some cases have malignant histological features and yet resolve spontaneously.

Metastasis

The eye and orbit are frequently sites for metastatic spread from distant malignancies. Tumours of the lung, breast, gastrointestinal tract, kidney and prostate are common sources.

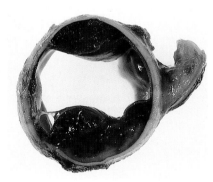

Fig. 3 **Choroidal melanoma.**

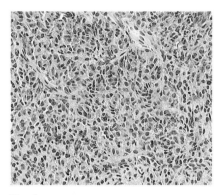

Fig. 4 **A pigmented choroidal melanoma of mixed cell type** (intermediate prognosis).

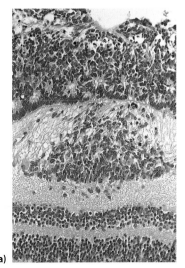

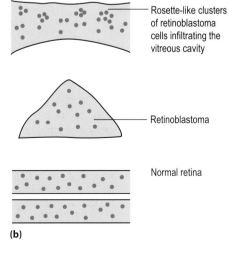

Rosette-like clusters of retinoblastoma cells infiltrating the vitreous cavity

Retinoblastoma

Normal retina

(a) **(b)**

Fig. 5 **Retinoblastoma.**

> *Ocular pathology*
>
> - Visual function depends on the maintenance off clear media.
> - Inflammation from any cause (trauma, infection, autoimmunity) disrupts the carefully controlled ocular environment crucial for normal vision.
> - Normal processes of repair and regeneration may be destructive and impair visual function.
> - Histological examination is necessary to confirm the clinical diagnosis of most lumps in and around the eye and orbit.
> - Orbital biopsy is hazardous.
> - The eye and orbit may be invaded by tumours from the lung, breast, gastrointestinal tract, kidney and prostate.

Ocular microbiology

Most infections of the eye (conjunctivitis and infection of the eyelid) are trivial, but severe infections of the globe and ocular adnexae are potentially sight-threatening and their progression may even present a threat to the patient's life (Table 1). Infective keratitis can progress to perforation or intraocular infection (endophthalmitis), but even after complete resolution scarring can severely impair sight. Orbital cellulitus may be complicated by meningitis or intracranial sinus thrombosis.

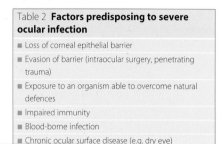

Table 1 Consequences of ocular infection

Depend on the infecting organism and the tissue involved
- Conjunctiva
  - loss of tear-producing glands
  - shrinkage (e.g. cicatricial entropion)
- Cornea
  - opacification
  - necrosis, even perforation
- Intraocular
  - retinal damage
  - structural disorganisation and blindness (phthisis)
- Orbital or even distant spread

Table 2 Factors predisposing to severe ocular infection

- Loss of corneal epithelial barrier
- Evasion of barrier (intraocular surgery, penetrating trauma)
- Exposure to an organism able to overcome natural defences
- Impaired immunity
- Blood-borne infection
- Chronic ocular surface disease (e.g. dry eye)

External ocular barriers to infection

Complex defences have evolved to prevent pathogenic microorganisms gaining access to the internal ocular and orbital tissues via the outer eye, whilst maintaining the controlled environment necessary for light transmission and refraction (Fig. 1).

The intact epithelial surfaces of the cornea and conjunctiva act as a substantial obstacle to pathogens, so acute or chronic disruption renders the eyes vulnerable (Table 2). The cornea's acute sensitivity to mechanical stimulation helps to prevent even trivial damage. The tear film serves to wash away potentially injurious agents, and several of its constituents have a direct antimicrobial action. These include the proteins lysozyme and lactoferrin, IgA, lymphocytes and cells of the monocyte–macrophage system.

Blinking, as well as clearing debris and microorganisms and distributing tears evenly, provides a rapid physical barrier in response to stimuli such as a visual or auditory threat.

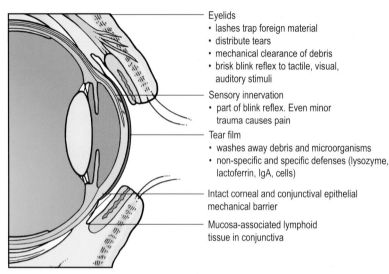

Eyelids
- lashes trap foreign material
- distribute tears
- mechanical clearance of debris
- brisk blink reflex to tactile, visual, auditory stimuli

Sensory innervation
- part of blink reflex. Even minor trauma causes pain

Tear film
- washes away debris and microorganisms
- non-specific and specific defenses (lysozyme, lactoferrin, IgA, cells)

Intact corneal and conjunctival epithelial mechanical barrier

Mucosa-associated lymphoid tissue in conjunctiva

Fig. 1 **External ocular barriers to infection.**

Normal flora of the external eye

A number of bacteria and other microorganisms are commensals of the lids and conjunctiva.

Staphylococcus epidermidis is the most common bacterium found on the normal periocular skin. *Staphylococcus aureus* is present less frequently. *Propionibacterium acnes* is common, as are a variety of fungi.

Organisms found on the conjunctiva of normal subjects include *Corynebacterium xerosis*, Neisseriae, Moraxella, staphylococci and streptococci.

Established infection

There are many factors which determine whether or not exposure to a particular microorganism will lead to infection. These include the number and virulence of the organism, and the integrity and effectiveness of the host defences.

Bacterial commensals are especially likely to be pathogenic when mechanical barriers are disrupted (e.g. corneal abrasion, intraocular surgery). *Neisseria gonorrhoeae* can penetrate the intact corneal epithelium. Viruses readily enter cells, and some, such as herpes simplex, may establish latency. Trachoma is a recurrent infection of a compromised ocular surface by *Chlamydia trachomatis*, resulting in lid, conjunctival and corneal scarring.

Obtaining specimens for laboratory investigation

The external eye is easily accessible, but collection of intraocular samples may be hazardous (Fig. 2). When an unusual infectious agent is suspected, and for all serious infections, it is essential to discuss the case with a medical microbiologist before taking samples. It is not possible to culture the pathogenic organism in all cases, despite the collection of an adequate sample.

Conjunctival swab

A sterile cotton-tipped probe is swept through the lower conjunctival fornix, taking care to avoid the lid margin and lashes (Fig. 3). The probe is used to inoculate culture medium. Samples can also be taken using special swabs and transport media for viruses and chlamydia, though culture of these can be unreliable and time-consuming and is no longer the method of first choice for diagnosis.

Conjunctival scrape

A topically anaesthetised conjunctival surface (usually the everted upper lid) is firmly scraped using a sterile spatula and the sample spread onto one (marked) side of a glass slide. Gram

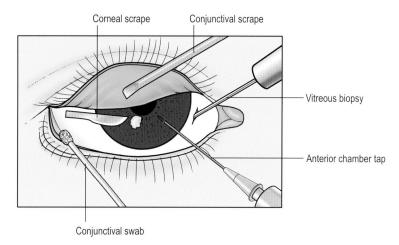

Fig. 2 **Techniques for obtaining specimens from the eye for microscopy and culture.**

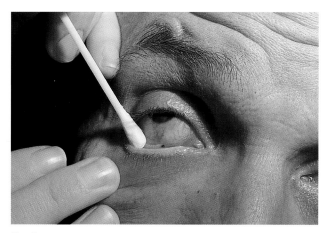

Fig. 3 **Taking a conjunctival swab.**

Table 3 **Culture media commonly used in ocular microbiology**	
Medium	**Organism**
Blood agar	Most aerobic bacteria and fungi
Chocolate agar	Aerobes (especially *Haemophilus influenzae*)
Sabouraud agar	Fungi
Escherichia coli-seeded agar	Acanthamoeba
Sodium chloride agar	Staphylococci
Cooked meat broth (e.g. Robertson's)	Anaerobes

staining of the sample can be used to identify bacterial class. Giemsa staining provides information regarding the cytological inflammatory response and may help identify inclusion bodies such as those found in chlamydial conjunctivitis. Other staining methods including immunodiagnostic techniques may be used to demonstrate particular organisms.

Corneal scrape

If necessary, a speculum is inserted to hold the eyelids apart. The eye is anaesthetised with a topical preparation and, under slit lamp observation, a spatula or disposable blade is used to obtain material from the base of a corneal ulcer. Microscopy and culture are arranged. Because of the sight-threatening nature of a corneal ulcer, it is essential that a range of culture media is inoculated (Table 3).

Anterior chamber tap

In a case of infective endophthalmitis a needle may be passed into the anterior chamber and a sample of aqueous humour withdrawn for microscopy and culture. The procedure has a low yield.

Vitreous biopsy

The definitive investigation in infective endophthalmitis is the microscopy and culture of a specimen of vitreous obtained using a cutting probe. In addition to conventional analysis, samples can be examined for evidence of microorganisms using the highly sensitive polymerase chain reaction (PCR) technique to amplify tiny quantities of DNA.

Serology

In some clinical situations, such as primary viral infection and chlamydial conjunctivitis, it is possible to detect rising antibody titres which can be diagnostic. In many other situations serology is unhelpful, including most cases of suspected toxoplasma retinochoroiditis.

Blood cultures are sometimes indicated, for instance if an endogenous aetiology is suspected (orbital cellulitis, endophthalmitis).

Antimicrobial therapy in ophthalmology

The basic principles of antimicrobial therapy are applicable to ophthalmology as in other medical specialties. Samples for diagnosis should generally be taken before beginning treatment. A frequent exception is simple bacterial or viral conjunctivitis in an adult, when a broad-spectrum antibiotic eye drop is prescribed.

Prophylactic antibiotics are routinely used following intraocular surgery and minor trauma, because of the relative difficulty of treating intraocular infection and because of the high level of functional impairment which may follow infection.

Ocular antimicrobial therapy can be administered topically (generally as drops or ointment), by subconjunctival or periocular/orbital injection, by injection directly into the vitreous cavity, or systemically. Many preparations penetrate the cornea well, and adequate drug levels in the aqueous can be achieved. However, most antibiotics fail to reach the vitreous, whether given locally or systemically, so direct intravitreal injection may be necessary to treat posterior segment infection.

Ocular microbiology

- Non-specific barriers to infection: lids and lashes, blinking, tear flow, epithelium.

- Specific barriers to infection: antibacterial tear constituents, immunity.

- The periocular skin and the conjunctiva are populated by commensal organisms which may cause disease.

- Special techniques permit samples to be obtained from various tissues of the eye for microscopy and culture.

- External infections may resolve spontaneously or respond rapidly to topical therapy.

- Intraocular infection may progress rapidly and cause irreversible loss of vision by the direct effects of the infecting organism and as a result of the host inflammatory response.

Ocular pharmacology

The effective administration of drugs to the eye presents unique advantages and challenges. The eye is one of the few organs to which therapeutic agents can be administered directly by noninvasive methods, but its interior is isolated from the circulation by substantial physiological barriers.

Methods of drug delivery

Topical
This is the most common route in ophthalmic practice. Despite its convenience, compliance is still a problem. There are several other disadvantages (Table 1).

The main route by which a topically administered drug reaches the anterior chamber is via the cornea (Fig. 1). Fat-soluble but not water-soluble drugs readily penetrate the corneal epithelium, whereas water solubility is required to cross the corneal stroma. The endothelium presents only a minor barrier. A drug is therefore best absorbed if it is both lipid- and water-soluble. 'Pro-drug' forms are sometimes used: a well-absorbed but inactive drug is converted to a more active form after absorption.

The two forms of topical preparation in common use are drops and ointment. Their contrasting properties are described in Table 2. Gels formulated using high molecular weight polymers overcome some of the disadvantages of conventional vehicles. Other methods of delivery such as membrane-regulated release systems and drug-saturated soft contact lenses are occasionally used, but are expensive and may be poorly tolerated.

Systemic
Systemic delivery is used much less frequently for the administration of ophthalmic drugs than the topical route. Physiological barriers prevent the penetration of systemically administered drugs into the eye in therapeutic concentrations.

For example, even with high plasma levels most antibacterial agents reach the vitreous in concentrations well below the therapeutic range (although in an inflamed eye penetration may be greater). Properties favouring ocular absorption of a systemically administered drug include high lipid solubility and low molecular weight.

Periocular/ocular injection
Drugs can be injected into the tissues surrounding the eye and, under some circumstances, directly into the globe itself. Orbital injection of local anaesthesia for surgery is routine. Injection of depot steroid into the orbit may be used to treat ocular inflammatory disorders. Topical treatment may be supplemented by subconjunctival injection, e.g. in the management of acute anterior uveitis or bacterial keratitis.

The treatment of intraocular bacterial infection frequently involves the injection of antibiotics directly into the globe. Slow release intravitreal systems are being developed in order to avoid the need for repeated injection to maintain adequate vitreous concentrations. This may have particular application in the treatment of chronic infection, such as cytomegalovirus retinitis in AIDS.

Adverse effects of systemic drugs on the eye
Drugs administered systemically for the treatment of non-ocular conditions may result in ocular side-effects (Table 3). Steroid-related cataract, common with long-term treatment, is a well-known example. The risk of ocular side-effects is rarely great and is usually outweighed by clinical therapeutic necessity.

Drugs used in ophthalmology
Important examples of drugs from each of the groups used in ophthalmology are listed in Table 4 together with their modes of action and adverse effects. Common or clinically important adverse effects only are listed. All drugs may cause an allergic reaction; the more likely agents are listed.

Table 1 Disadvantages of the topical route of administration

- Elderly and disabled patients may be unable to handle dropper bottles
- Some preparations cause stinging/blurring
- Vitreous penetration is generally poor
- Drug vehicle can act as a culture medium for contaminant microorganisms
- Preservatives are usually necessary and may provoke allergic or toxic reactions
- Limited compatibility with contact lens wear
- Systemic absorption and adverse effects still occur

Table 2 Contrasting properties of eye drops and ointment

	Drops	Ointment
Visual effect of vehicle	Minimal	Significant blurring
Drug–eye contact time	Relatively short	Relatively long
Peak tear concentration	High	Low
Contact lens wear	Avoid soft lenses (unless preservative-free)	Incompatible
Ease of use	Dependent on container	Can be messy and awkward

Table 3 Adverse effects of systemic drugs on the eye

Drug	Ocular side effect
Amiodarone	Corneal deposits (vortex keratopathy)
Antiepileptics	Ocular motility dysfunction
Trihexyphenidyl, benzatropine, atropine	Pupillary dilation (risk of angle closure glaucoma)
Corticosteroids	Cataract, glaucoma
Digitalis	Abnormal colour vision
Ethambutol, quinine	Optic neuropathy
Hydroxychloroquine, chloroquine	Retinal degeneration change ('bull's eye' macula), corneal deposits
Opiates	Pupillary constriction
Phenothiazines	Retinal oedema, pigmentary retinopathy, ocular motility dysfunction
Sulphonamides, NSAIDs	Stevens–Johnson syndrome
Tamoxifen	Pigmentary retinopathy
Vigabatrin	Visual field defects

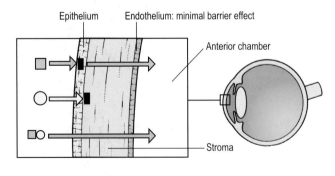

Epithelium   Endothelium: minimal barrier effect

Anterior chamber

Stroma

☐ Hydrophilic molecule cannot penetrate epithelium

◯ Lipophilic molecule cannot penetrate stroma

☐◯ Molecule with hydro- and lipophilic properties is readily absorbed

Fig. 1 **Drug absorption via the cornea.**

Table 4 **Summary of drugs commonly used in ophthalmology**

	Examples in common use	Mode of administration	Action	Side-effects
Glaucoma treatment (note that different types of glaucoma may require different therapeutic approaches)	Beta-blockers; timolol, carteolol, betaxolol, levobunolol	Topical	Reduce aqueous secretion by inhibitory action on beta-adrenoceptors in the ciliary body	Ocular: irritation Systemic: bronchospasm, bradycardia, exacerbation of heart failure, nightmares
	Muscarinic (parasympathetic) stimulants: pilocarpine	Topical	Increase aqueous outflow via trabecular meshwork by ciliary muscle contraction	Ocular: miosis (reduced vision in presence of cataract, retinal examination impaired), spasm of accommodation, brow ache Systemic: sweating, bradycardia, gastrointestinal disturbance
	Alpha2-stimulants: brimonidine, apraclonidine	Topical	Reduce aqueous secretion by selective stimulation of alpha2- and adrenoceptors in the ciliary body increase outflow by uveoscleral route	Ocular: allergy, mydriasis, eyelid retraction Systemic: dry mouth, hypotension, drowsiness, headache
	Prostaglandin derivatives: latanoprost, travoprost, bimatoprost, unoprostone	Topical	Increase aqueous outflow by the uveoscleral route	Ocular: iris darkening, conjunctival hyperaemia, eyelash growth Systemic: bitter taste, asthma
	Carbonic anhydrase inhibitors	Systemic (acetazolamide), topical (dorzolamide, brinzolamide)	Reduce aqueous secretion by the ciliary body	Ocular route: irritation, allergy Systemic (generally systemic use): malaise, paraesthesia, urea and electrolyte disturbance, aplastic anaemia
Mydriatics and cycloplegics (for retinal examination and objective refraction (retinoscopy)	Antimuscarinics: tropicamide, cyclopentolate, atropine	Topical	Inhibit muscarinic receptors of parasympathetic nervous system to paralyse pupillary sphincter and ciliary muscle	Ocular: blurred vision (especially for near), glare, angle closure glaucoma Systemic: tachycardia, dry mouth, confusion, tremor
	Alpha-stimulant: phenylephrine	Topical	Stimulates dilator muscle of the pupil; no cycloplegic effect	Ocular: blurred vision, glare, angle closure glaucoma, conjunctival blanching Systemic: hypertension
Lubricants A range of preparations is available for the treatment of dry eyes	Carbomers, hypromellose, polyvinyl alcohol, liquid paraffin	Topical	Exact mechanism depends on agent	Ocular: preservative allergy/toxicity, blurred vision (especially ointments) ointments)
Anti-inflammatory agents Most important drugs in this category are corticosteroids; a variety of other agents is available, including systemic immunosuppressants	Corticosteroids: prednisolone, betamethasone, dexamethasone	Topical, periocular injection, systemic	Suppression of broad spectrum of inflammatory processes	Ocular: glaucoma (especially with local administration), cataract (especially prolonged systemic use), exacerbation of some infections e.g. herpes simplex Systemic: negligible with topical use; common and varied with systemic administration
	Mast cell stabilisers (cromoglicate, nedocromil, lodoxamide)	Topical	Stabilise mast cells	Ocular: irritation
	Antihistamines	Topical (antazoline, azelastine, levocabastine), systemic (chlorphenamine, terfenadine, cetirizine)	Block histamine receptor (azelastine also stabilises most cells)	Ocular route: irritation Systemic route: drowsiness
	Non-steroidal anti-inflammatory drugs: systemic help to control ocular pain and inflammation; topical increasingly used for pain of corneal abrasion, for inflammation after cataract surgery, and to maintain pupil dilation during cataract surgery	Topical (ketorolac, diclofenac, flurbiprofen)	Modulate prostaglandin production	Systemic: peptic ulceration, asthma
Anti-infective agents Topically applied antibacterial and antiviral drugs are very commonly prescribed; the use of antifungal and antiparasitic agents is much less frequent	Antibacterials: chloramphenicol, gentamicin, ciprofloxacin, neomycin, fusidic acid	Topical, occasionally intra-ocular, systemic	Range of activities and specificities	Vary with agent Ocular: allergy; corneal toxicity common with intensive use Systemic: generally only with systemic use
	Antivirals: aciclovir	Topical, systemic, intravitreal	Inhibits herpes virus DNA synthesis	Ocular: blurred vision, corneal toxicity Systemic: rashes; kidney, liver and other effects may occur with systemic use
Local anaesthetics Major uses are to relieve pain and thereby assist with clinical examination, and the facilitation of surgical anaesthesia	Oxybuprocaine, proxymetacaine, tetracaine, lidocaine	Topical, periocular injection	Block conduction along nerve fibres	Ocular: irritation, corneal toxicity Systemic: generally accidental intravascular or intrathecal (cerebrospinal fluid) injection during surgical anaesthesia: cardiac arrhythmias, respiratory depression
Botulinum toxin: used in the management of certain ocular motility disorders and blepharospasm, and to induce ptosis for corneal protection		Injection at site of action	Prevents release of the neurotransmitter acetylcholine at neuromuscular junctions	Dependent on treatment site: e.g. unwanted ptosis or double vision

Diseases

Eyelids: blepharitis, dermatitis and lumps

Blepharitis

Blepharitis (Fig. 1) is a common disorder of the lids which may cause persistent and annoying symptoms of irritation, watering and redness. The signs are often minimal, yet symptoms may be severe. There are two main varieties: staphylococcal and seborrhoeic.

Staphylococcal blepharitis

This is primarily due to infection of the lid margins by staphylococcal bacteria (*aureus* and *epidermidis*). The lid margin is inflamed and coated with scales. The lashes are stuck together by crusts.

Seborrhoeic blepharitis

This variant can occur in association with seborrhoeic dermatitis. The abnormality is an overproduction of sebum by glands at the lid margin (especially the meibomian glands). Bacteria metabolise the sebum, producing irritant free fatty acids. The lid margin is less inflamed than in staphylococcal blepharitis. Careful examination will show plugs of sebum in the meibomian gland orifices (Fig. 2) and a foamy tear film.

Both types of blepharitis frequently overlap and may be indistinguishable from each other. Both can give rise to a secondary conjunctivitis, which may not be infective, and to punctate corneal epithelial erosions, seen after instillation of fluorescein and examination with a blue light.

Other associations include:

- disturbance of the tear film ('dry eye')
- corneal scarring and vascularisation, especially of the inferior cornea
- peripheral corneal ulceration and infiltration
- eyelash abnormalities, such as inward growth (trichiasis), whitening and loss
- stye (external hordeolum, a bacterial eyelash folliculitis) (Fig. 3)
- internal hordeolum (acute bacterial meibomian gland infection)
- chalazion (meibomian gland lipogranuloma) (Fig. 4)
- acne rosacea (erythema, pustules, hypertrophic sebaceous glands, rhinophyma).

Management

This is directed against the presence of scales, crusts and sebum; against bacterial infection of the lid margins; and to supplement tear inadequacy.

Treatments include:

- **Lid hygiene**. Cotton-tipped buds, cotton wool balls or a soft cloth soaked in warm water are used to rub away scales, crusts and sebum, to reduce the bacterial load and to express plugged meibomian glands.
- **Antibiotics**. Topical antibiotic ointments (e.g. chloramphenicol) cling to the lid margin better than drops. Systemic antibiotics (tetracycline, doxycycline), for 6–12 weeks at a time, may be used in severe or persistent cases.

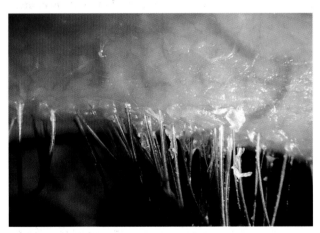

Fig. 1 **Blepharitis: eyelash crusts.**

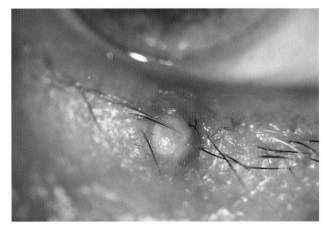

Fig. 3 **A stye.**

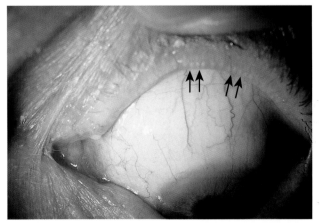

Fig. 2 **Blepharitis: meibomian gland disease.**

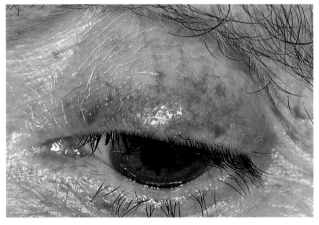

Fig. 4 **A chalazion.**

Table 1 Eyelid lumps

Type	Description	Treatment
Infections		
Of eyelash (stye)	Staphylococcal abscess discharging at lash exit	Antibiotic ointment, warm compresses
Of meibomian gland	Staphylococcal abscess pointing through lid skin or conjunctiva	Antibiotic ointment, warm compresses
Molluscum contagiosum	Viral umbilicated nodule causing chronic conjunctivitis	Express, cauterise or excise
Viral warts	Papillomatous	Leave or excise
Inflammation		
Chalazion	Slowly enlarging chronic granuloma of meibomian gland	Leave or incise and curette
Retention cysts		
Of Möll (sweat gland)	Thin-walled lid margin cyst containing clear fluid	Leave or marsupialise
Of Zeis (sebaceous gland)	Sebum-containing lid margin cyst	Leave or excise
Sebaceous	Sebum-containing cyst	Leave or excise
Benign tumours		
Papilloma	Sessile or pedunculated nodule	Leave or excise
Seborrhoeic keratosis	Greasy brown with friable surface	Leave or excise
Senile keratosis	Flat, scaly, multiple; may transform into a squamous cell carcinoma	Leave or excise
Xanthelasma	Lipid-containing deposit	Leave or excise
Keratoacanthoma	Keratin-filled crater which usually regresses	Leave or excise
Cutaneous horn	Keratinised outgrowth which may overlie a BCC	Remove
Haemangioma	Strawberry-like tumour of infancy which grows and then regresses entirely by age 5 years	Await regression, unless visual development threatened
Naevus	Pigmented	Leave
Malignant tumours		
Basal cell carcinoma (BCC)	Nodular, ulcerative or ill-defined sclerosing types; locally invasive	Complete excision; radiotherapy and cryotherapy less effective
Squamous cell carcinoma	Much less common than BCC; rapidly growing nodule, ulcer or papilloma which may metastasise	Complete excision
Sebaceous gland carcinoma	Very rare, arising from a meibomian gland; may mimic recurrent chalazion	Complete excision
Melanoma	Rare pigmented tumour which may be spreading or nodular	Complete excision

■ **Artifical tear drops**. These give considerable relief, and should be administered on an 'as often as necessary' basis. There are many types available. Patients may need to try several before finding the one that suits them best.

Acute infection (external or internal hordeolum) is helped by warm compresses. If severe, especially if there is associated cellulitis, surgical drainage and systemic antibiotic use may be required.

It should be emphasised to patients that the condition is chronic and relapsing–remitting, and that it may not be possible to effect a complete cure. Relief of symptoms depends on good motivation and regular treatment, particularly lid hygiene.

Dermatitis

The eyelids are susceptible to allergic disease. The skin is thin and only loosely attached to the underlying tissues. For these reasons, only low doses of allergen may be needed to produce severe changes.

Contact dermatitis can be caused by make-up, skin cleansers, hair shampoos and sprays, and anything that might be transferred to the eyelids on fingers. Features include erythema, swelling and scales of the eyelid skin (Fig. 5). Medications administered to the eyes may be the fault, and will cause an associated conjunctivitis. The dermatitis will extend down onto the cheek, where the medication spills out.

Atopic individuals can develop periocular dermatitis and conjunctivitis. The chronic nature of the conjunctivitis may lead to permanent corneal changes.

Eyelid lumps

These are common and varied. Acute infective lesions have the typical features of infection: pain, swelling, inflammation and purulent discharge. The sterile chalazion is also very common. Differentiation from other eyelid swellings is usually easy (Table 1).

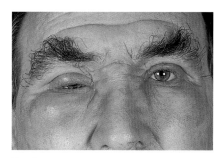

Fig. 5 **Contact dermatitis due to chloramphenicol drops.**

Management depends both on the clinical diagnosis and on patient expectation. Many obviously benign lesions such as retention cysts can safely be left alone, but patients often request their removal. Malignancies, the most common being the basal cell carcinoma (Fig. 6), need to be managed aggressively.

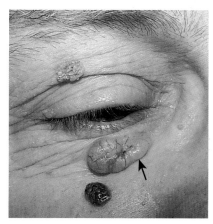

Fig. 6 **A basal cell carcinoma on the lower eyelid.**

Eyelids: blepharitis, dermatitis and lumps

Blepharitis

■ a common cause of irritable, red, sticky eyes

■ signs may be slight in comparison with the symptoms

■ management is lid hygiene, antibiotics and artificial tears.

Dermatitis

■ usually allergic (contact dermatitis) or in association with eczema.

Eyelid swellings

■ differentiate between infection/inflammation, retention cysts and benign and malignant tumours.

Eyelids: abnormalities of position

Abnormal position of the eyelids is common. The term ptosis describes a droopy upper eyelid which, when severe, may interfere with vision. Entropion (turning inwards) and ectropion (turning outwards) both cause watering, as a result of eyelashes irritating the ocular surface (entropion) or impairment of tear collection by the eyelid puncta (ectropion).

Ptosis

Ptosis (Fig. 1) may be unilateral or bilateral, and may be asymmetrical. Remember that the upper lid is lifted by contraction of levator muscle (third cranial nerve (Fig. 2), plus sympathetic innervation of a smooth muscle component), and that the lids are closed by orbicularis oculi (facial nerve). A facial nerve palsy does not cause a ptosis.

The normally positioned upper eyelid covers the upper 1–2 mm of the cornea. In ptosis, the upper eyelid margin lies below this level.

Differential diagnosis

Asymmetry of lid position may occur without ptosis. A sunken eye (enophthalmos), which may follow orbital wall fracture, can mimic a ptosis. A proptosed or large eye may give the appearance of ptosis in the normal fellow eye. In dermatochalasis there is an excess of upper lid skin, which may hang below the lid margin.

Causes

These include:

- involutional (ageing) changes
- third nerve palsy
- myasthenia gravis
- trauma to the levator muscle
- Horner's syndrome
- mitochondrial myopathies.

Age-related loss of the connections between the levator muscle and the eyelid skin is common and usually bilateral. The ptosis may be sufficient to impair vision, particularly of the upper field.

A third nerve palsy will have other features, including a divergent squint and sometimes a dilated pupil. Important causes of a third nerve palsy include atherosclerosis, diabetes mellitus and, rarely but importantly, an expanding intracranial aneurysm.

Myasthenia gravis, in which antibodies to the acetylcholine receptor in the neuromuscular junction prevent normal muscle depolarisation and contraction, may present with ocular signs only, before the onset of systemic disease features. Typically the ptosis is variable, becoming worse with effort, and therefore worse at the end of the day. There may also be abnormal eye movements, causing double vision.

Trauma to the upper eyelid may break the connections between the levator muscle and the eyelid skin.

In Horner's syndrome, the sympathetic innervation of Muller's muscle, a smooth muscle component of levator, is disrupted. This may occur at any point along the course of the sympathetic pathway though important sites include the brainstem (in association with other neurological signs) and in the neck, particularly due to invasive lung cancer. The ptosis will be accompanied by a small pupil and sometimes by dryness and flushing of facial skin on the affected side.

Mitochondrial myopathies are rare but interesting disorders, since they are transmitted by mitochondrial DNA, which is acquired from the mother not the father. Retinal pigmentation,

resembling retinitis pigmentosa, and cardiac conduction anomalies may occur.

Ptosis may be congenital or acquired. Although any of the above causes may result in a congenital ptosis, this is usually idiopathic or part of a congenital Horner's syndrome.

Patient assessment

First confirm the presence of a true ptosis, and then establish whether this is congenital or acquired. Old photographs may help. Compensatory contraction of frontalis muscle, which has some attachment to the upper lid, causes wrinkling of the forehead (Fig. 1). An overacting frontalis muscle should be neutralised by firmly pressing against the brow to prevent transference of the contracting force from the forehead to the lid. This will show the severity and may reveal a bilateral ptosis. The skin crease is high or absent in involutional ptosis. Other signs (third nerve palsy, myasthenia, Horner's syndrome) should be sought.

Management

This depends very much on the cause. Surgical restoration of the connections between levator and the eyelid skin is commonly performed for involutional ptosis. Myasthenia is managed with cholinesterase inhibitors (increasing the availability of acetylcholine) and immunosuppressants. However, any other procedure to lift the upper lid risks exposing the cornea, so surgical intervention may not be advisable. Ptosis props, wire scaffolds which fasten to spectacle frames and push the lid upwards, may be all that is required. Elevation of the lid in a third nerve palsy may produce disabling double vision.

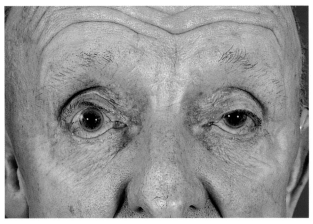

Fig. 1 **Ptosis** (left eye).

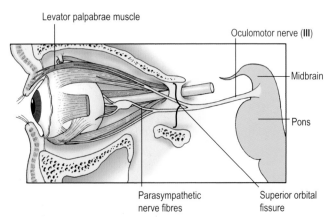

Levator palpabrae muscle

Oculomotor nerve (**III**)

Midbrain

Pons

Parasympathetic nerve fibres

Superior orbital fissure

Fig. 2 **Nerve supply to levator muscle.**

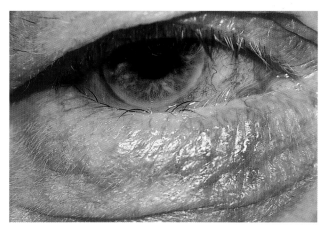

Fig. 3 **Entropion.**

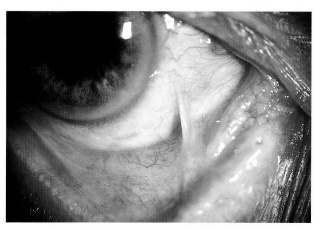

Fig. 4 **Conjunctival scarring.**

Entropion

Entropion (Fig. 3) is a turning inwards of the lid margin such that normal eyelashes abrade the eyeball. Entropion may affect the upper or lower eyelid. In the UK, upper lid entropion is rare, but worldwide it is more common, due to the contractile scarring process which occurs in trachoma.

Causes
These include:

- involutional (ageing) changes
- conjunctival scarring (cicatricial)
- spasm of orbicularis oculi.

Lower eyelid position is the result of a balance between several forces, particularly the inwardly directed orbicularis oculi muscle and the outwardly pulling lower lid retractors. This balance is upset in involutional entropion.

Any conjunctival scarring process may result in entropion. Chief among these are alkali burns, trachoma and Stevens–Johnson syndrome. Pull the eyelid away from the eyeball to look for adhesions across the conjunctival fornix (Fig. 4).

Spasm of orbicularis may be primary, often with hemifacial spasm, or secondary, usually due to persistent ocular irritation.

Ocular consequences
The inwardly turning lid causes the eyelashes to rub against the eyeball, resulting in foreign body-type sensation and reflex watering. The abrasive action of the eyelashes may cause a corneal abrasion with risk of bacterial corneal infection. Corneal ulceration requires urgent ophthalmological referral.

Management
Most cases are managed with a simple surgical procedure, although conjunctival scarring is very hard to overcome. Blepharospasm can be treated with repeated injections of botulinum toxin.

Ectropion

Ectropion (Fig. 5) is a turning outwards of the eyelid margin. Causes include:

- involutional (ageing) changes
- facial nerve palsy
- eyelid skin scarring (cicatricial)
- bulky eyelid tumours.

Just as involutional changes may cause entropion, so they may also lead to ectropion. Whilst a facial nerve palsy does not result in a droopy upper lid, it does cause an ectropion. Any scarring process involving facial skin or bulky eyelid tumours can cause the lower lid to turn outwards.

Ocular consequences
Ectropion almost always affects the lower eyelid. The main consequence is watering, since the normal collection of tears into the punctum is impaired. The exposed lid conjunctiva may become inflamed and keratinised. Corneal exposure may result from an extreme ectropion; ulceration requires urgent specialist referral.

Management
Involutional ectropion can be corrected by a simple surgical procedure. If the cause is a facial nerve palsy, then the likelihood of recovery of nerve function should be considered. If recovery is likely, frequent administration of lubricating ointment may be sufficient, but if the cornea is at risk, a temporary lateral tarsorrhaphy (in which the eyelids are sutured together) should be performed or botulinum toxin injected to induce a protective ptosis. Permanent facial nerve palsy and cicatricial ectropion are managed surgically.

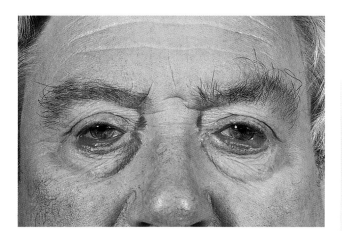

Fig. 5 **Ectropion.**

Eyelids: abnormalities of position

- Ptosis:
  - consider aetiology: congenital vs acquired
  - main causes are ageing changes, third nerve palsy, myasthenia gravis and Horner's syndrome.
- Entropion:
  - usually due to ageing changes in the eyelid, but look for conjunctival scarring
  - check the cornea – ulceration requires urgent referral.
- Ectropion:
  - usually due to ageing changes or facial nerve palsy
  - check the cornea – ulceration requires urgent referral.

Tear secretion and drainage

Adequate ocular lubrication is required in the maintenance of corneal health, both as a barrier to infection and as an optical medium. Disturbance of the balance between production and drainage of tears impairs these functions.

The dry eye

Aetiopathogenesis

Dry eye syndrome can result from a deficiency in any one of the three components of the tear film, namely the outer lipid, the middle aqueous and the inner mucin layers.

Aqueous tear deficiency, or keratoconjunctivitis sicca, is an uncommon but severe cause of dry eyes. The aqueous layer smooths the optical interface, washes away debris and conveys oxygen and antibacterial elements to the corneal and conjunctival surfaces. Approximately 95% of the aqueous component is secreted by the main lacrimal gland, situated in the anterolateral orbit, with additional secretion by accessory glands in the conjunctiva.

Lacrimal gland dysfunction is usually caused by inflammation, especially autoimmune, but other causes include scarring of the secretory ducts and excision of the gland. Pure keratoconjunctivitis sicca involves the lacrimal gland alone, but if the salivary and other glands are involved in an autoimmune process the term 'primary Sjögren's syndrome' is used. Secondary Sjögren's syndrome is found as part of a systemic autoimmune disorder such as rheumatoid arthritis.

The inner mucinous layer, produced mainly by conjunctival goblet cells, provides a hydrophilic attachment for the aqueous component. Mucin deficiency, also known as xerophthalmia, occurs when large numbers of goblet cells are damaged by extensive conjunctival scarring (alkali burn, cicatrising conjunctival disease). Hypovitaminosis A is another cause of inadequate mucin production.

Disturbance of the lipid layer is usually found as a component of blepharitis.

Clinical features

Pure aqueous deficiency is unusual, but poor tear film quality is common and is especially associated with blepharitis, the signs of which may be trivial. The chief symptom is persistent irritation, often with a feeling of dryness.

Identification of the clinical signs requires slit lamp examination and the instillation of a dye such as fluorescein or rose bengal. Fluorescein mixes into the tears, permitting qualitative examination of the tear film, and stains punctate epithelial erosions in the cornea and conjunctiva. Mucus strands and debris may also be seen. Schirmer's test (Fig. 1), which measures the wetting of a strip of filter paper, is an objective but unreliable test. Severe dry eye can result in corneal epithelial loss, scarring and vascularisation. Corneal thinning (melt) and perforation are rare consequences (Fig. 2).

Patient assessment should include systemic enquiry for evidence of rheumatoid arthritis and dryness of other mucosal surfaces.

Management

Treatment options include:

- conservative measures such as the humidification of room air, the attachment of side-pieces to spectacles (both measures reduce tear evaporation)
- tear supplements: a variety are available and all may need to be tried in the search for comfort
- lacrimal punctal occlusion – temporary (e.g. silicone plugs, Fig. 3) or permanent (cautery).

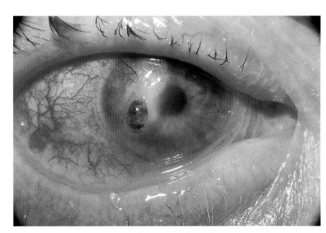

Fig. 2 **Corneal melt in a patient with rheumatoid arthritis.**

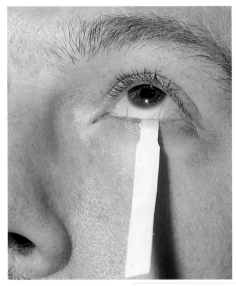

Fig. 1 **Schirmer's test.**

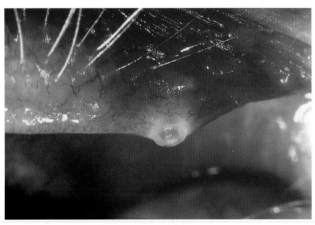

Fig. 3 **A silicone plug in the right upper punctum.**

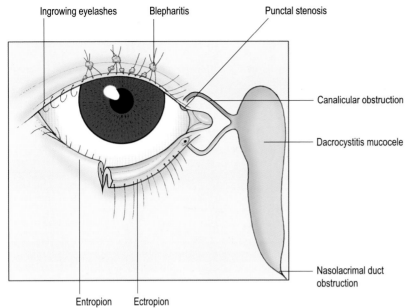

Ingrowing eyelashes Blepharitis Punctal stenosis

Canalicular obstruction

Dacrocystitis mucocele

Nasolacrimal duct obstruction

Entropion Ectropion

Fig. 4 **The watering eye.**

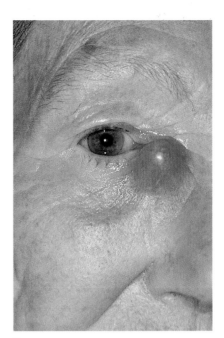

Fig. 5 **Acute dacrocystitis.**

Blepharitis should be managed by regular lid hygiene, to restore meibomian gland function, and with antibiotics. Toxicity to preservative in drops and difficulties with handling bottles, particularly in patients with rheumatoid arthritis, are common problems and can limit the efficacy of tear substitutes.

The watering eye

Aetiopathogenesis

Inappropriate watering of the eye can be due to failure of the lacrimal drainage system (epiphora) or to oversecretion of tears (lacrimation) (Fig. 4).

Inadequate drainage can be caused by obstruction or can result from failure of the lacrimal pump, the physiological mechanism which propels tears into the lacrimal sac. Pump failure is usually due to facial nerve palsy or to ectropion.

Obstruction may be congenital or acquired. Congenital obstruction usually results from a failure of complete development of the nasolacrimal duct, which may continue to develop in infancy leading to spontaneous resolution. Acquired obstruction may occur at any point along the drainage pathway, though obstruction of the distal nasolacrimal duct by involutional changes is most common.

Oversecretion of tears follows ocular irritation by eyelashes and even, paradoxically, as a reflex to the ocular irritation that accompanies blepharitis and dry eye states.

Patient assessment

The most important task is to differentiate between oversecretion and drainage failure. Careful examination of the eyelids and eyeball should identify causes of oversecretion. Nasolacrimal duct obstruction may lead to the formation of a mucocele, a non-infected swelling of the lacrimal sac, or to a lacrimal sac infection, dacrocystitis (Fig. 5). Both appear as swellings at the medial canthus. The contents of a mucocele may be expressed into the conjunctival fornix by digital pressure. Acute dacrocystitis is a tender, red swelling, often with a purulent point of discharge.

After instillation of anaesthetic drops, gentle probing using a cannula attached to a syringe of saline solution may localise an obstruction. Punctal stenosis will prevent

insertion of the cannula. If a canaliculus is blocked, the cannula cannot be passed into the sac. If the sac can be entered, regurgitation of injected saline solution indicates duct obstruction. Sometimes the saline solution passes into the nasopharynx, where it is tasted. This may indicate partial obstruction or functional drainage failure.

Occasionally a dacrocystogram (injection of radio-opaque dye into the system) is helpful. Dacroscintillography uses a radioisotope and gamma camera to assess physiological flow. The drainage passages can be visualised directly using a tiny fibreoptic probe.

Treatment

Treatment is aimed at the cause, though overcoming functional drainage failure may not be possible. Blepharitis and dry eye states should be treated. Ingrowing eyelashes, entropion and ectropion require a surgical approach.

If congenital nasolacrimal duct obstruction fails to resolve spontaneously by the age of about 9 months, probing the system under general anaesthesia is usually curative. Acquired nasolacrimal duct obstruction may require a bypass procedure (dacrocystorhinostomy), linking the sac to the nasal cavity by removal of intervening bone. This is a major operation, so evaluation of patient health and the severity of symptoms is necessary.

Creation of a bypass channel with an endonasal laser is an increasingly popular option. Although the results are less reliable than the open procedure, this technique is quicker and can be performed under local anaesthesia as a day case.

> ## Tear secretion and drainage
>
> **Dry eye**
> - usually poor quality tears associated with blepharitis
> - often significant symptoms but minimal signs
> - tear substitutes used frequently are main therapy.
>
> **Watering eye**
> - caused by excessive production (look for ocular irritation) or inadequate drainage, usually due to nasolacrimal duct obstruction.

Orbital diseases

Although a wide range of diseases can affect the orbit, these share many common features, by occupying volume within a confined space and by damaging specific orbital structures (Fig. 1). Therefore, the main clinical features of orbital disease are not specific to the underlying pathology.

Clinical features

The chief features are proptosis, visual loss, double vision and pain.

Proptosis is displacement forwards of the eye caused by a space-occupying effect. Lesions behind the eyeball push the eye directly forwards (axial proptosis); lesions elsewhere push the globe off axis (non-axial proptosis) (Fig. 2).

Visual loss is usually caused by a compressive effect on the optic nerve. Visual acuity, colour vision and peripheral vision may all be affected. The optic disc may be swollen or atrophic.

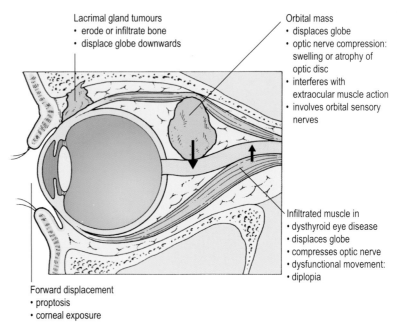

Lacrimal gland tumours
- erode or infiltrate bone
- displace globe downwards

Orbital mass
- displaces globe
- optic nerve compression: swelling or atrophy of optic disc
- interferes with extraocular muscle action
- involves orbital sensory nerves

Infiltrated muscle in
- dysthyroid eye disease
- displaces globe
- compresses optic nerve
- dysfunctional movement:
- diplopia

Forward displacement
- proptosis
- corneal exposure

Fig. 1 **Mechanisms for the development of the clinical features of orbital disease.**

Double vision (diplopia) may occur if the two eyes are misaligned in straight ahead gaze or become misaligned during movement. Displacement of the eye or involvement of the motor nerves or extraocular muscles in the disease process may be responsible.

Pain is frequently present. It may occur as a result of a space-occupying effect or through involvement of sensory nerves.

Patient assessment

A complete history and examination generally produces a short list of differential diagnoses, but further investigation is usually essential. Chief amongst these are CT and MRI scanning.

Diseases

Thyroid eye disease

Ocular complications of disorders of the thyroid gland are common and may even precede the development of biochemical thyroid dysfunction. Usually the association is with a hyperactive gland (Graves' disease or Graves' ophthalmopathy), but hypo- and even euthyroid states may

occur. The clinical features are caused by infiltration of the orbital tissues by inflammatory cells and oedema, since the underlying pathogenesis is a humoral and cell-mediated autoimmunity to orbital antigens. Consequently, there are two phases to the clinical course: an initial acute inflammatory phase lasting two or three years during which symptoms and signs change frequently, followed by a stable chronic phase.

Proptosis and double vision are the main problems. Proptosis, which may be unilateral, is more than a cosmetic nuisance, because corneal exposure leading to visual loss may result. The double vision is often variable in time and severity. Lid retraction produces a 'staring' appearance (Fig. 3). Lid lag, the jerky downwards movement of the upper lid on downgaze, also occurs. Visual loss may result from optic nerve compression.

Treatments for thyroid eye disease include:

- lubrication
- double vision: prisms attached to spectacles (though these may need to be changed frequently); sometimes surgery
- eyelid surgery to overcome lid retraction
- systemic immunosuppression (e.g. steroids), orbital radiotherapy and surgical orbital decompression (fracturing the walls of the orbit to allow displacement of orbital contents) for severe proptosis and optic nerve compression.

Treatment of underlying thyroid dysfunction does not influence the course of the ocular disease.

Orbital cellulitis

Infection within the orbit is usually associated with infection in a paranasal sinus. In addition to proptosis and reduced ocular movement, there is redness and swelling of the eyelids and conjunctival injection (Fig. 4). There may be systemic signs of infection, such as pyrexia and malaise. Causative organisms include *Haemoaphilus influenzae* (especially in young children), *Streptococcus pneumoniae* and anaerobes. Orbital cellulitis may be rapidly progressive and needs to be

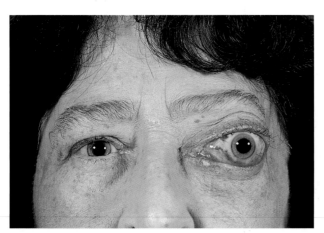

Fig. 2 **Non-axial proptosis.**

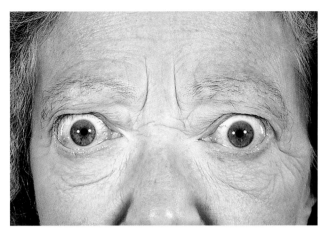

Fig. 3 **The starting eyes of dysthyroid eye disease.**

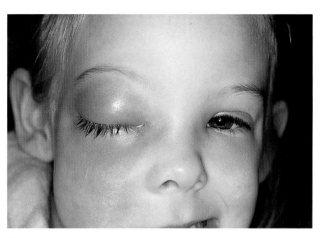

Fig. 4 **Orbital cellutitis.**

treated aggressively if visual loss and intracranial spread are to be prevented. Appropriate intravenous antibiotics should be started immediately. Failure to respond despite treatment may indicate the development of an orbital abscess, seen on CT scan.

Trauma

The orbital rim protects the globe against major blunt trauma, but squash balls and other objects which fit within the rim push the eyeball backwards causing a sudden increase in intraorbital pressure. This pressure is transmitted to the thin floor of the orbit which may fracture. (Occasionally the medial wall may fracture.) Once the initial haematoma subsides, the eye is seen to be displaced backwards (enophthalmos). Entrapment of orbital tissues within the fracture site leads to double vision, especially on up- and downgaze. Damage to the infraorbital nerve alters sensation on the cheek.

Systemic antibiotics should be prescribed for what is, in effect, a compound fracture. Surgical management is controversial. Some authorities advise early surgery to free entrapped tissues from the fracture site, but ocular movement will often improve without intervention.

Tumours

Any orbital structure may give rise to a primary benign or malignant tumour, and the orbit may be involved in secondary spread from adjacent or distant sites.

- **Primary tumours** of most importance are: cavernous haemangioma; meningiomas (Fig. 5), especially of the sphenoid bone or optic nerve sheath; benign and malignant tumours of the lacrimal gland; and lymphoma.

- **Secondary tumours** can spread from various sources including the lung, the breast and the prostate gland.

Several tumours have a predilection for children.

- **Dermoid cysts** are swellings at the upper nasal or temporal aspects of the anterior orbit.
- **Capillary haemangiomas** develop soon after birth. They may be confined to the orbit, but may show on the upper lid as a strawberry naevus. They regress spontaneously, usually by school age, but treatment (e.g. local steroids) may be necessary to prevent amblyopia.
- **Optic nerve gliomas** cause early visual loss and often occur in association with neurofibromatosis.
- **Rhabdomyosarcoma** may rarely mimic orbital cellulitis.

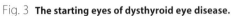

Fig. 5 **CT scan of the head: a meningioma with involvement of the lateral wall of the orbit.**

Vascular abnormalities

Orbital varix is a congenital venous abnormality but may not present until early adulthood. Proptosis is intermittent and related to posture and straining. Carotico–cavernous fistula is a communication between the internal carotid artery and the cavernous sinus. It occurs suddenly, as a result of trauma or spontaneously, typically in the elderly. The pulsatile proptosis is associated with a loud bruit, haemorrhagic conjunctival swelling and dilated episcleral vessels.

Idiopathic inflammatory disorders

Idiopathic inflammation ('pseudotumour') may occur in the orbital soft tissues, at the orbital apex or in an extraocular muscle. Pain is a common symptom. Clinical features depend on the location of the inflammatory focus: at the orbital apex, there will be axial proptosis and optic nerve compression; extraocular muscle involvement (orbital myositis) may cause proptosis and strabismus with double vision upon movement of the eye towards or away from the affected muscle.

Orbital diseases

Main clinical features of disease
- proptosis or enophthalmos
- reduced visual acuity, loss of colour vision, field loss, optic disc swelling or pallor
- double vision
- pain.

Main causes of disease
- thyroid eye disease
- orbital cellulitis
- trauma
- tumours
- vascular abnormalities.

Conjunctiva: infective inflammation

The term conjunctivitis describes any form of conjunctival inflammation (Fig. 1), but usually refers to bacterial or viral infection.

Bacterial conjunctivitis

A variety of microorganisms may infect the conjunctiva (Table 1).

Bacterial conjunctivitis manifests as a sticky red eye of acute onset, generally associated with mild to moderate itching, burning or grittiness and little or no effect on vision. Although one eye only may be involved at first, the fellow eye is usually affected after a short delay. There may be a history of contact with conjunctivitis.

Lid swelling, conjunctival hyperaemia and purulent discharge are prominent (Fig. 2). Papillae (Fig. 3, Table 2) give the conjunctiva a velvet-like appearance. Corneal ulceration should be excluded as the cause of the red eye. The pupil should be round and normally reactive. The discharge may cause mild blurring of vision, but if the visual acuity is more than mildly reduced, corneal involvement or an alternative, more serious, diagnosis should be suspected.

Management

Most bacterial conjunctivitis is self-limiting, settling spontaneously in a few days even without treatment and does not require investigation. However, the prescription of a broad-spectrum topical antibiotic such as chloramphenicol, gentamicin or fusidic acid is usual.

If the infection fails to respond to the initial choice of topical antibiotic, a conjunctival swab sent for microscopy and culture can be helpful, but a viral cause is more likely. Atypical features or a particularly severe or persistent infection warrant referral to an ophthalmologist.

Conjunctival infection with *Neisseria gonorrhoeae* produces an especially acute and severe clinical picture. Unlike most other bacteria, *N. gonorrhoeae* can penetrate the intact corneal epithelium and cause corneal infection (keratitis). Management includes identification of the organism and intensive specific antibiotic therapy.

Conjunctivitis often accompanies blepharitis, which also requires treatment.

Chlamydial infections

Chlamydia, usually regarded as very small bacteria, are obligate intracellular pathogens.

Inclusion conjunctivitis

This sexually transmitted infection is caused by serotypes D–K of *Chlamydia trachomatis* and characteristically presents in young adults as an acute or subacute follicular conjunctivitis clinically similar to a viral infection (Fig. 4, Table 2). Urethral or vaginal symptoms may occur. Microscopy, immunofluorescence and culture of conjunctival scrapes aid diagnosis.

Treatment is with oral antibiotics: tetracycline or erythromycin. Systemic assessment and contact tracing is managed by a genitourinary physician.

Infection in the neonate requires systemic erythromycin; tetracycline is unsuitable because of discoloration of growing teeth. Mother and contacts should also be investigated and treated.

Trachoma

Serotypes A–C of *Chlamydia trachomatis* cause trachoma, a chronic conjunctivitis endemic to areas with inadequate sanitary facilities in many developing countries. The infection follows a chronic course leading to severe conjunctival cicatricial change with entropion, trichiasis, dry eye and secondary corneal ulceration and scarring. It is the third most common cause of blindness worldwide. Diagnosis and treatment is similar to chlamydial inclusion conjunctivitis

Viral conjunctivitis

The viruses most commonly causing conjunctivitis are listed in Table 1, but conjunctival involvement can also occur in the course of the systemic childhood viral infections, including measles and chicken pox. Symptomatically, viral conjunctivitis is similar to the bacterial form but the predominant discharge is watery rather than purulent, although

Table 1 **Infectious agents commonly causing conjunctivitis**
Bacterial
■ *Staphylococcus aureus*
■ *Staphylococcus epidermidis*
■ *Streptococcus pneumoniae*
■ *Haemophilus influenzae*
■ *Neisseria gonorrhoeae* (esp. in neonates)
■ *Chlamydia trachomatis*
Viruses
■ Adenoviruses (multiple serotypes)
■ Herpes viruses

Table 2 **Papillae and follicles**	Papillae	Follicles
Appearance	Fine to 'giant' focal, irregular flattened conjunctival elevations enclosing vascular core	Opalescent ovoid elevations similar to tiny grains of rice; vessels surrounding rather than within follicles
Structure	Hyperplastic epithelium enclosing vascular tuft, chronic inflammatory infiltrate	Foci of hyperplastic lymphoid tissue
Common causes	Bacterial conjunctivitis, allergic conjunctivitis, contact lens wear, chronic conjunctivitis of any cause	Viral and chlamydial conjunctivitis, acute allergic conjunctivitis

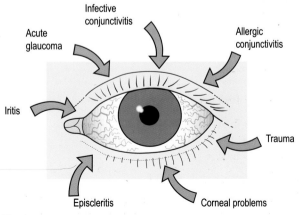

Fig. 1 **Causes of red eye.**

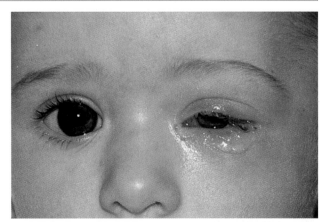

Fig. 2 **Bacterial conjunctivitis.**

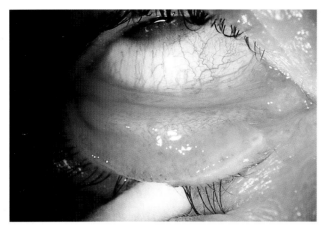

Fig. 3 **Conjunctival papillae.**

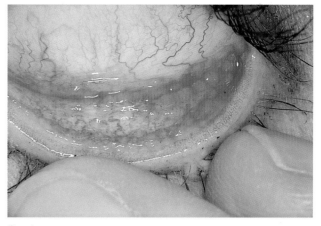

Fig. 4 **Conjunctival follicles.**

night-time discharge causes the eyelids to be sticky in the morning. Unilateral progressing to bilateral involvement and moderate grittiness are typical. Non-specific systemic symptoms with pyrexia and an upper respiratory tract infection commonly occur at the same time.

Examination confirms a watery discharge, conjunctival hyperaemia and, frequently, petechial conjunctival haemorrhages. In contrast to the papillae of bacterial infection, follicles (resembling grains of rice) are the major conjunctival feature (Fig. 4, Table 2). Punctate corneal epithelial erosions are frequent. Corneal ulceration, such as the dendritic lesion of herpes simplex keratitis, should be excluded. Microscopic subepithelial corneal infiltrates may develop under the epithelial erosions and result in glare, which can persist following resolution of the acute conjunctivitis (Fig. 5). Secondary iritis may occasionally occur, particularly in association with a severe episode or with herpes simplex infection.

Pre-auricular lymph node enlargement is frequently present. There may be severe eyelid swelling sufficient to close the lids altogether. This swelling occasionally extends down the face towards the ear.

Conjunctivitis caused by primary or secondary herpes simplex virus infection can occur, usually accompanied by a vesicular rash on the eyelid skin. Primary infection, however, is often subclinical. Ophthalmic shingles can cause conjunctivitis; the characteristic skin changes may be mild and easily overlooked.

A follicular conjunctivitis may also be caused by viral particles shed from the lesion of molluscum contagiosum, a tiny whitish papillomatous lump on the eyelid margin that is easily treated by curettage.

Viral infection usually settles within about two weeks without treatment. Symptoms of irritation, redness and stickiness after sleep may occasionally persist for months.

In refractory cases, investigation by means of conjunctival swabs and scrapes is indicated. This may identify an alternative microorganism (such as chlamydia) or may suggest a distinct inflammatory process.

Management

Specific treatment is not available for the majority of cases of viral conjunctivitis, although topical antiviral agents including aciclovir and trifluorothymidine are effective against herpes simplex.

Vasoconstrictor/antihistamine combinations may reduce symptoms. Topical antibiotics may have some merit as prophylaxis against secondary bacterial infection, and artificial tears are sometimes used for their soothing effect. Topical steroids effectively reduce symptoms, but should only be used in cases where the diagnosis is certain and under ophthalmological supervision.

Adenoviral conjunctivitis may cause epidemic infection. Simple measures including personal hygiene and avoidance of contact should be practised.

Neonatal conjunctivitis

Neonatal conjunctivitis is common. Onset within the first few hours of birth is usually chemically induced. Thereafter, *Chlamydia trachomatis* and other bacteria are likely causes. Rapidly progressive disease suggests more severe infection, such as *Neisseria gonorrhoeae*. Corneal examination is mandatory.

Congenital glaucoma and congenital nasolacrimal duct obstruction may mimic conjunctivitis.

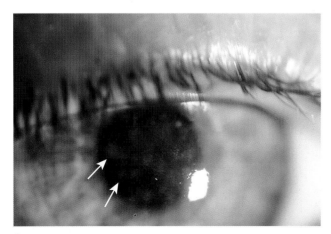

Fig. 5 **Adenoviral keratitis.**

Conjunctiva: infective inflammation

Bacterial conjunctivitis
- Causes red eyes with a purulent discharge.
- Usually responds quickly to a broad-spectrum topical antibiotic.
- Papillae may be evident.

Viral conjunctivitis
- Most common cause is adenovirus.
- Causes red eyes with a watery discharge.
- Follicles are prominent.
- No specific treatment is available in most cases.

Chlamydia trachomatis
- Range of serotypes cause sexually transmitted infection, with conjunctivitis that may be persistent unless treated.
- Causes blinding trachoma in developing countries.

Conjunctiva: non-infective inflammation

Allergic conjunctivitis

Acute allergic conjunctivitis

Acute allergic conjunctivitis has a rapid onset. Chief features are itching, lid swelling and conjunctival oedema (chemosis) (Fig. 1). It is most frequently seen in children following exposure to pollen or some other allergen that has been inoculated into the conjunctival fornices. The reaction settles spontaneously in a few hours. An acute allergic reaction can also occur in response to the administration of topical eye medication, though in this situation the signs tend to resemble a contact dermatitis with variable skin erythema and excoriation.

Seasonal and perennial allergic conjunctivitis

Seasonal allergic conjunctivitis refers to the mild to moderate itching, redness and watering that occur in association with hay fever at times of a high environmental pollen count. Mucous discharge and conjunctival papillae are seen. Perennial allergic conjunctivitis, caused by allergens other than pollen (such as the house dust mite), is clinically similar but tends not to have a seasonal pattern.

Treatment

Immediate relief is achieved with the use of a topical vasoconstrictor/ antihistamine preparation. Topical antihistamines such as levocabastine can be very effective. Systemic antihistamines such as terfenadine can be used acutely and prophylactically. Topical sodium cromoglicate and related agents (page 23) stabilise mast cells, reducing the response to allergen. They cannot treat acute disease but are effective prophylactically. Severe cases may warrant treatment with weak topical steroids under ophthalmological supervision.

Chronic allergic conjunctivitis

The terms 'vernal' and 'atopic' keratoconjunctivitis refer to a spectrum of chronic allergic conjunctivitis, usually occurring in atopic individuals. Vernal occurs in children, atopic in adults. Both are caused by repeated exposure to allergen in association with immune system dysfunction (Fig. 2). Seasonal exacerbations are frequently a feature. Symptoms consist of itching, burning, grittiness and redness of both eyes. There is a stringy mucous discharge and large, even 'giant', conjunctival papillae, particularly under the upper lids (Fig. 3). Ulceration and infiltration of the upper part of the cornea is a feature of vernal keratoconjunctivitis. Treatment is similar to that of seasonal allergic conjunctivitis, though topical steroids are more often required.

Giant papillary conjunctivitis is an allergic response to a foreign body, especially hard and soft contact lenses. The upper lid conjunctiva has a 'cobblestone' appearance (Fig. 3). Removal of the foreign body is usually sufficient treatment.

Cicatricial conjunctivitis and bullous disorders

Erythema multiforme is a cutaneous reaction pattern associated with circulating immune complexes. Stevens–Johnson syndrome or erythema multiforme major denotes severe disease involving the skin and the oral and conjunctival mucous membranes. Those most often affected are young adults. The disease may be idiopathic or may be a response to a variety of infections or to drugs such as sulphonamides and salicylates. Mortality is significant.

Symptoms include malaise, arthralgia, skin rash and redness of the eyes and mouth. The characteristic 'target' skin lesions are bullae into which haemorrhage has occurred. The oral mucosa and lips become erythematous and crusted.

Bilateral moderate to severe conjunctivitis is common, with bullae and necrotic patches progressing to extensive conjunctival scarring.

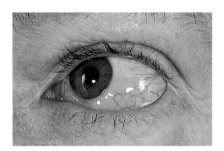

Fig. 1 **Conjunctival chemosis in acute allergic conjunctivitis.**

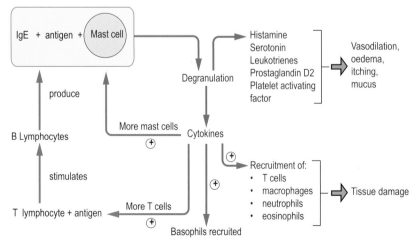

Fig. 2 **The pathogenesis of chronic allergic disease.**

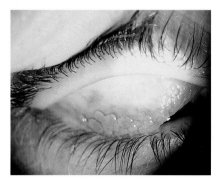

Fig. 3 **Giant papillae.**

Ocular cicatricial pemphigoid

This is a chronic relapsing/remitting inflammatory disorder of the conjunctiva which results in shrinkage (cicatrisation). Mucous membranes at other sites may also be involved. Vesicles and erythematous plaques in the skin arise in a minority. Patients tend to be female and in later middle age. Ocular cicatricial pemphigoid is thought to represent one end of a spectrum of bullous disorders.

Ocular symptoms are typically sub-acute, with bilateral redness, grittiness and watering in the earlier stages. Hyperaemia, papillae and bullae are followed by contraction of the conjunctival fornices (Fig. 4).

Both Stevens–Johnson syndrome and cicatricial pemphigoid may result in severe mechanical abnormalities of the lids including entropion and trichiasis, with secondary corneal scarring that may eventually lead to blindness (Fig. 5). Loss of conjunctival glands leads to dry eye. Tear drainage may be impaired. Ocular treatment consists of adequate tear replacement, topical steroids and treatment of infection. Dapsone may be effective. Other forms of systemic immunosuppression are sometimes tried.

Surgery is performed for lid abnormalities where these are contributing to ocular damage, but manipulation of the conjunctiva may precipitate an increase in inflammation. Penetrating keratoplasty for corneal scarring carries a poor prognosis. Surgical insertion of a prosthetic cornea (keratoprosthesis) may offer the only chance of restoring sight in advanced disease.

Conjunctival cicatrisation may also follow prolonged topical treatment, particularly with adrenaline and pilocarpine. Pemphigus vulgaris and epidermolysis bullosa may also involve the conjuctiva.

Superior limbic keratoconjunctivitis

This disorder, affecting the upper conjunctiva and cornea, may be a feature of thyroid eye disease. There is injection of the superior bulbar conjunctiva and vascularisation of the adjacent limbus. The upper lid conjunctiva develops papillae. A filamentary keratitis affects the upper third of the cornea (Fig. 6, Table 1). (Filaments are strands of epithelium and mucus that attach to pinpoint defects in the epithelium.)

Treatment with artificial tears and topical steroids is of little benefit. Acetylcysteine drops may reduce the number of filaments. Spontaneous resolution eventually occurs, but only after a long period.

Table 1 **Diseases that feature corneal filaments (strands of mucus attached to the epithelium)**
Keratoconjunctivitis sicca
Recurrent corneal erosion syndrome
Corneal anaesthesia
Herpes simplex keratitis
Superior limbic keratoconjunctivitis

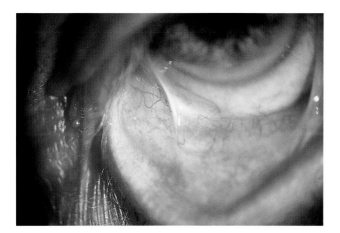

Fig. 4 **Conjunctival contraction.**

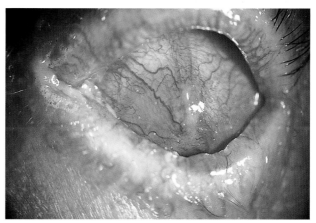

Fig. 5 **Corneal scarring secondary to severe conjunctival contraction.**

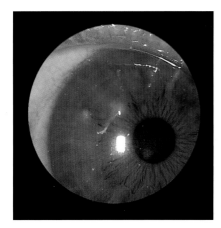

Fig. 6 **Filamentary keratitis.**

Conjunctiva: non-infective inflammation

- Acute allergic conjunctivitis is episodic and settles without treatment.
- Seasonal allergic conjunctivitis varies from mild to severe.
- Chronic forms of allergic conjunctivitis:
  – vernal keratoconjunctivitis, sometimes with corneal ulceration, in children
  – atopic keratoconjunctivitis runs a prolonged course in atopic adults
  – symptoms may be severe and difficult to treat.
- Stevens–Johnson syndrome is an acute systemic vasculitis which can be fatal; an ophthalmology opinion is essential.
- Ocular cicatricial pemphigoid is a chronic autoimmune inflammation causing conjunctival contraction and secondary corneal damage.
- Superior limbic keratoconjunctivitis is associated with thyroid eye disease. Signs are restricted to superior bulbar conjunctiva, superior limbus and upper third of the cornea.

Cornea: inflammation

The cornea may be affected by inflammation (keratitis) with or without an infective component. This is followed by tissue repair, with scarring and vascularisation, which may result in corneal opacification and astigmatism and, therefore, severe visual loss.

Viral infection

Herpes simplex virus

Infection may be primary or secondary. Primary infection usually occurs subclinically in childhood but can cause a blepharoconjunctivitis and a dendritic type of corneal ulcer. A latent stage in the trigeminal ganglion may be followed by reactivation, in which virus travels along the nerve to the eye. Typical corneal involvement is the dendritic ulcer, so-called because of its branching pattern (Fig. 1). Ulcers may be multiple.

If the infection is confined to the epithelium, healing occurs without scarring. However, stromal inflammation may occur and is always followed by some degree of scarring. There may also be an anterior uveitis.

Many patients also suffer from recurrent cutaneous infection ('cold sores').

It is important to confirm the diagnosis by identification of virus from cells scraped from the ulcer edge, particularly because infection may be recurrent and may mimic many other types of corneal infection and inflammation.

Ulceration will resolve spontaneously, though it is usual to administer aciclovir ointment. The treatment of stromal disease and anterior uveitis may require careful topical steroid use, usually after healing of any epithelial disease. Topical steroids applied to a herpetic corneal ulcer will result in an amoeboid ulcer, which is slow to heal and very hard to treat.

Varicella-zoster virus

Primary infection (chicken pox) may cause a conjunctivitis and, rarely, a dendritic ulcer. Secondary infection, or shingles, resulting from latent virus in the trigeminal ganglion, may affect any ocular or adnexal structure.

Ophthalmic involvement (herpes zoster ophthalmicus, or HZO) accounts for about 10% of cases of shingles. Any of the three divisions of the trigeminal nerve may be affected, but the first (ophthalmic) division is most common. The skin rash is typical (Fig. 2): it is dermatomal, involving the forehead to occiput and the upper lid, tending to spare the lower lid but usually affecting the side of the nose, which is supplied by nerve fibres that course through the orbit.

Conjunctivitis is usual. Keratitis and anterior uveitis with a secondary glaucoma are common. The keratitis principally affects the stroma, though dendritic and non-dendritic ulceration may occur. Scleritis and epicleritis are frequent problems.

Conjunctivitis and iritis may continue for many months, but the most disabling sequelae are recurrent keratitis with scarring and post-herpetic neuralgia, which may continue for years.

Systemic aciclovir is of proven benefit in early ophthalmic shingles, reducing the duration and severity of the acute disease as well as the post-herpetic neuralgia. Topical steroids have a significant role in suppressing ocular inflammation but may lead to 'dependence', in which inflammation returns as soon as steroid use is discontinued.

Adenovirus

Adenoviral conjunctivitis is very common. In a minority, a keratitis, consisting of multiple faint fluffy white opacities, may occur These cause blurring of vision, glare (see Fig. 5, p. 35), photophobia and grittiness. Topical steroids dramatically improve symptoms but should only be administered if herpetic keratitis can be excluded.

Bacterial infection

The corneal epithelium is an effective barrier against the entry of micro-organisms into the eye.

Predisposing factors which make it possible for bacteria to reach the stroma include:

- corneal trauma
- contact lens wear
- a chronically compromised ocular surface, such as dry eye, blepharitis and bullous keratopathy (endothelial failure)
- herpetic keratitis
- corneal exposure (facial nerve palsy, proptosis)
- corneal anaesthesia (neurotrophic keratopathy)
- immunosuppression, including topical steroid use.

The contact lens wearer with redness and discomfort should be carefully examined for the presence of corneal infection and referred for further assessment by an ophthalmologist. Bacterial keratitis is usually obvious (Fig. 3). There is a purulent conjunctivitis, a corneal ulcer and a corneal opacity. Vision is reduced. Bacterial corneal infection can progress to intraocular infection (endophthalmitis), leading to blindness. Intraocular infection is suggested by the presence of white cells in the anterior chamber (a hypopyon, Fig. 3).

Common organisms are *Staphylococcus aureus* and *epidermidis*, *Streptococcus pneumoniae*, enterobacter (coliforms, *Proteus*, *Klebsiella*) and *Pseudomonas aeruginosa*. The last causes a particularly aggressive infection.

Unless a bacterial keratitis is mild, urgent investigation and admission for intensive treatment are mandatory. Conjunctival and corneal samples are sent for microscopy and culture. Broad-spectrum topical antibiotics, such as a quinolone, are administered frequently 24 hours per day, initially, until a favourable response is seen. Predisposing factors that can be modified should also be treated.

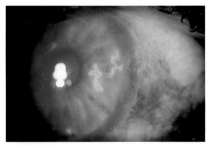

Fig. 1 **Corneal dendritic ulceration resulting from secondary herpes simplex virus infection.**

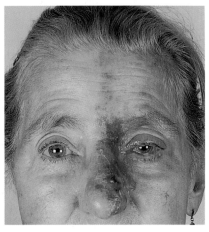

Fig. 2 **Ophthalmic shingles.**

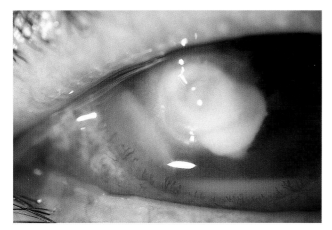

Fig. 3 **Bacterial keratitis with a hypopyon.**

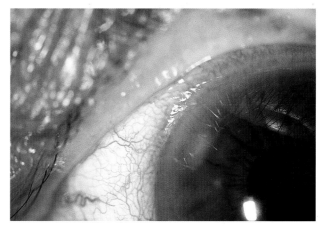

Fig. 4 **Marginal keratitis.**

Sometimes subconjunctival and systemic antibiotics are also prescribed.

Despite the likelihood of permanent scarring, topical steroids are used only when resolution of the infective element of the inflammation is thought to have occurred.

Protozoan infection

Corneal infection by the protozoan *Acanthamoeba* is increasing in incidence. It is an ubiquitous organism present even in tap water. Keratitis is usually severe and unrelenting and does not respond to standard antibiotic treatment. It is particularly associated with contact lens use and can grow in many of the solutions used in contact lens care. Typically there is pain disproportionate to the ocular signs, and stromal keratitis without ulceration. The diagnosis is difficult and is often missed. Treatment with appropriate agents is prolonged.

Peripheral corneal thinning

Thinning (or melting) of the cornea adjacent to and usually parallel to the limbus may occur with or without epithelial loss (ulceration) and with or without inflammation. Progressive thinning can lead to corneal perforation and intraocular infection, or to severe astigmatism. The long term prognosis for patients with a corneal melt associated with a systemic disease is poor.

Non-autoimmune causes

Marginal keratitis

Blepharitis, which may occur in isolation or with acne rosacea, is a common cause of marginal corneal ulceration (Fig. 4). Marginal keratitis is usually a sterile hypersensitivity reaction to bacterial toxins. Topical steroids and antibiotics result in rapid resolution. The underlying disorder should also be treated (q.v.).

Infection

Exclude by appropriate investigation of corneal scrapes.

Dellen

A localised swelling of the conjunctiva, such as postsurgical inflammation or a pterygium, prevents normal transit of tears across the adjacent cornea, which becomes thinned as a result.

Autoimmune causes

Melting of the corneal stroma starts adjacent to the limbus and may proceed centrally and circumferentially. Epithelial loss need not be present.

Organ-specific disease

Primary Sjögren's syndrome causes dryness of mucous membranes, particularly the conjunctiva and the mouth. Painless melting may begin insidiously and progress inexorably. Mooren's ulcer is a rare painful progressive melting process that results in marked astigmatism.

Generalised disease

Rheumatoid arthritis causes a secondary Sjögren's syndrome. Systemic lupus erythematosus, Wegener's granulomatosis and polyarteritis nodosa are rare recognised causes of corneal melting.

Management

Local therapy

This includes reversal of tear insufficiency by the frequent instillation of artificial tears and punctal occlusion, together with treatment of any infection.

Systemic therapy

Investigation and treatment of any underlying disorder is necessary, usually in conjunction with a rheumatologist or dermatologist.

Corneal surgery

Surgery may be indicated for a variety of reasons:

- Diagnostic biopsy.
- Corneal perforation.
- Superficial corneal scars: removed surgically (replaced by a layer of donor cornea – lamellar keratoplasty) or using the excimer laser (phototherapeutic keratectomy).
- Restoration of visual potential after dense scarring: full-thickness corneal transplantation (penetrating keratoplasty). Scarring as a result of herpes simplex infection is one of the main indications for corneal transplantation in the UK. However the prognosis in these eyes is less good than for other indications for transplantation, because of an increased risk of immune rejection.

Cornea: inflammation

- Infection
  - viral: herpes simplex and herpes zoster cause similar ocular signs and may mimic other corneal inflammations; adenoviral keratitis causes blurring and photophobia after viral conjunctivitis
  - bacterial: purulent conjunctivitis, infiltrated ulcer; immediate investigation and antibiotic treatment
  - *Acanthamoeba*: associated with contact lens use; fails to respond to standard antibiotic treatment.

- Ocular surface disease (trauma, dry eye, etc.) predisposes the cornea to penetration by microorganisms.

- Corneal melting or thinning may be caused by infection, reduction of tear flow or an autoimmune process associated with systemic disease.

Cornea: dystrophies and degenerations

A dystrophy is a primary intrinsic hereditary disorder, with bilateral manifestation. The term degeneration refers to changes occurring secondary to an insult in previously normal tissue and includes ageing. The changes need not be bilateral.

Only the more common disorders will be described.

Dystrophies

Recurrent corneal erosion syndrome

Many dystrophies and degenerations interfere with adhesion of the epithelium to its basement membrane, causing epithelial instability and breakdown.

Patients suffer a tendency to develop spontaneous corneal abrasions, typically awakening with a severe foreign body sensation in the affected eye. The eye is inflamed and waters profusely. Symptoms may improve during the day. Examination may show mild conjunctival injection only, punctate fluorescein staining or a corneal abrasion. Poor lid closure should be considered as a cause. Frequently a history of previous trauma is given. In other cases the underlying cause is a familial epithelial dystrophy such as the 'map-dot-fingerprint' pattern. Several dystrophies of the corneal stroma may also be associated with recurrent spontaneous abrasion.

Between episodes, the eye may appear normal, but tiny epithelial cysts or whorls may be seen on careful slit lamp examination.

Persistent daily discomfort should be treated with regular lubrication, especially at night. Epithelial loss is managed as for any corneal abrasion, with chloramphenicol ointment, a mydriatic and padding. Recurrent corneal erosion syndrome caused by trauma eventually resolves, but if symptoms are persistent, a soft bandage contact lens (without refractive power) may be used. Persistent cases with distressing symptoms might be helped by surgical intervention in the form of stromal needle puncture or excimer laser ablation (phototherapeutic keratectomy). These procedures help create a fibrous adhesion of the epithelium to the stroma.

Stromal dystrophies

In lattice dystrophy, amyloid is deposited in the corneal stroma in a branching pattern (Fig. 1). Inheritance is autosomal dominant. Patients present with symptoms of recurrent corneal erosion. The central cornea becomes clouded, leading to visual loss.

Other stromal dystrophies such as Reis–Bückler's dystrophy of the anterior stroma and granular and macular dystrophies occur less commonly. Vision may be affected to a variable extent in these conditions, and recurrent corneal erosion syndrome may occur.

If visual loss is significant, full-thickness corneal grafting (penetrating keratoplasty) (Fig. 2) is indicated.

Cornea guttata and Fuchs' endothelial dystrophy

Cornea guttata is a state of endothelial cell dysfunction or loss that occurs in the ageing cornea.

Progressive endothelial cell loss (Fuchs' dystrophy) may lead to decompensation, such that the cornea becomes oedematous, losing transparency and reducing vision. Painful epithelial blisters (bullous keratopathy) are typical. Scarring and vascularisation may also occur.

Eyes with endothelial dysfunction may decompensate following routine cataract surgery leading to aphakic and pseudophakic bullous keratopathy (Fig. 3).

Symptoms of discomfort and pain may be relieved by topical lubricants and hypertonic solutions such as 5% saline, which helps to dehydrate the cornea. Penetrating keratoplasty is performed for visual loss, and for pain, even when the visual prognosis is poor.

Keratoconus

Keratoconus is an acquired abnormality of corneal shape of gradual onset. It is usually bilateral but asymmetrical. The incidence is approximately 1 in 20 000. Systemic conditions such as Down and Marfan syndromes and ocular conditions such as atopic keratoconjunctivitis are associated.

The cornea protrudes forwards like a cone, the apex of which becomes thinned, scarred and distorted (Fig. 4). Patients

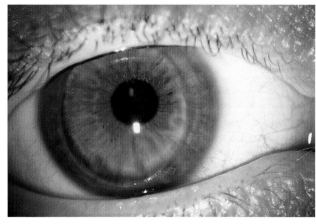

Fig. 2 **A corneal transplant** (penetrating keroplasty).

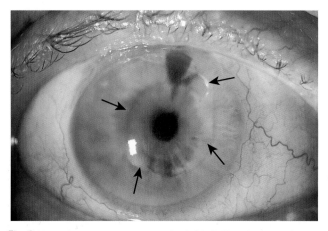

Fig. 3 **A semi-opaque cornea (pseudophakic bullous keratopathy).**
Note the anterior chamber lens implant (arrows).

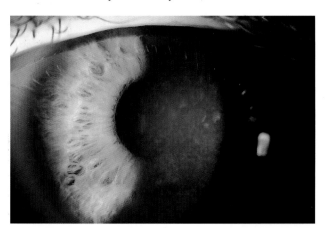

Fig. 1 **Lattice dystrophy.**

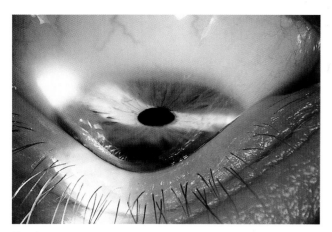

Fig. 4 **Keratoconus.**

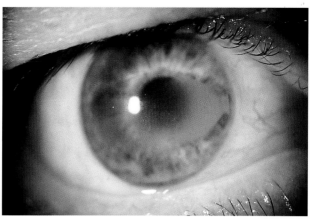

Fig. 6 **Band keratopathy.**

present with slow visual deterioration, often initially uniocular, owing to progressive myopia and astigmatism.

Acute hydrops may occur: the stroma suddenly becomes thickened and hazy as aqueous humour enters through splits in Desçemet's membrane, resulting in scarring.

Diagnosis depends on evidence of progressive myopic astigmatism and on identification of the many subtle changes seen on slit lamp microscopy. Computed corneal topography assists in early diagnosis.

Early management is aimed at refractive correction: contact lenses will usually achieve satisfactory vision when spectacles can no longer correct astigmatism. Acute hydrops is treated with lubricants and hypertonic solutions.

Penetrating keratoplasty is indicated when the refractive error becomes too extreme to be corrected by optical means, or when scarring has substantially decreased vision. The prognosis following transplantation is very good.

Degenerations

Pterygium

A pterygium is a non-neoplastic fibrovascular degenerative change that extends from the interpalpebral conjunctiva into the cornea beneath the epithelium (Fig. 5). Rarely it encroaches onto the visual axis or causes astigmatism. Often it is a cosmetic problem, or gives rise to a persistent foreign body sensation. Surgical removal is not straightforward since recurrence is common.

A pinguecula is a similar process involving the interpalpebral conjunctiva only, without growth onto the cornea. Surgery is not required.

Band keratopathy

Band keratopathy, in which there is subepithelial deposition of calcium in the interpalpebral region (Fig. 6), can arise

secondary to chronic intraocular inflammation or in association with systemic hypercalcaemia. It can also occur idiopathically in older patients. Symptoms include reduced vision due to involvement of the central cornea and a gritty sensation caused by irregularity of the overlying epithelium. If symptoms are significant, the calcium can be removed by local debridement.

Lipid deposition

The accumulation of discrete corneal lipid deposits is usually found adjacent to an area of corneal vascularisation, such as occurs after corneal infection.

Arcus senilis is a common degeneration present in most elderly people, consisting of a narrow circumferential strip of lipid laid down in the peripheral cornea. In young adults it may indicate hyperlipidaemia.

Salzmann nodular degeneration

A cornea exposed to chronic inflammation may develop whitish nodular. The overlying epithelium tends to be irregular and unstable, and lubricants are helpful in maintaining comfort.

Crystalline keratopathy

A variety of conditions can lead to the formation of tiny crystals within the cornea including dysproteinaemias, the therapeutic administration of gold and metabolic disease such as cystinosis and gout.

Vortex keratopathy

This is the epithelial deposition on a characteristically whorled pattern of some medications, chiefly amiodarone. It does not cause any symptom.

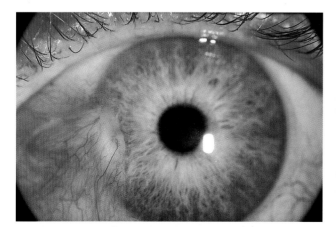

Fig. 5 **Pterygium.**

Cornea: dystrophies and degenerations

- Recurrent erosion syndrome is caused by an epithelial or stromal dystrophy or by previous trauma. Treat with regular lubrication, patching or bandage contact lens. Consider surgical intervention if persistent severe symptoms.

- Endothelial failure can be caused by ageing or cataract surgery. Progressive stromal oedema leads to loss of transparency and formation of epithelial bullae. It may require corneal transplantation.

- Keratoconus features progressive myopic astigmatism caused by distorted corneal shape. Treated with transplantation when optical treatment is insufficient.

- Pterygium is an interpalpebral fibrovascular growth which can be removed surgically.

- Band keratopathy, in which there is interpalpebral calcium deposition, may be associated with hypercalcaemia or chronic inflammation. Visual loss and pain are treated with debridement.

Glaucoma: primary open angle

The glaucomas are a mixed group of disorders that have some common features: optic disc cupping, visual field loss and, usually, raised intraocular pressure (IOP). Raised pressure without optic disc damage and visual field loss constitutes ocular hypertension; glaucoma in the absence of high pressure is known as normal, or low tension glaucoma. The glaucomas may be classified into:

- primary versus secondary
- open versus closed
- congenital versus acquired.

Acquired primary open angle glaucoma (POAG) is the most common type, affecting 1% of those aged over 40 years, and 10% of the over-80s. Untreated, it is usually a progressive disease.

Pathogenesis

Aqueous humour drains through the trabecular meshwork in the angle between the cornea and the iris. Over time this sieve-like structure undergoes morphological changes, the cause of which is not known, which impair drainage. The consequent rise in intraocular pressure is transmitted to the optic disc where nerve fibre damage occurs. However, elevated pressure is not the sole cause of damage, given the existence of ocular hypertension and normal tension glaucoma. It is likely that impairment of the optic nerve

blood supply or aspects of optic nerve head structure are important.

Risk factors

These include:

- genetic: more common in first-degree relatives
- increasing age
- diabetes mellitus
- myopia
- black race.

Clinical features

Primary open angle glaucoma does not cause any symptoms until it is so advanced that central vision is threatened. It does not present with headache or eye pain or with loss of visual acuity.

The chief signs are raised intraocular pressure, optic disc cupping and peripheral visual field loss.

Detection

Since only advanced disease may be symptomatic, detection depends on chance and on examination of at-risk individuals. Routine optometry examinations account for the majority of hospital referrals. Since first-degree relatives of glaucoma sufferers are considered to be at most risk, they are entitled to a free sight test. However, a national screening programme is not yet justified.

Examination

Intraocular pressure can be measured by a variety of techniques. The most reliable and accurate is performed at the slit lamp, using a corneal applanating prism after instillation of anaesthetic and fluorescein drops. Other methods include assessment of corneal resistance to a calibrated puff of air and an electronic applanator. Digital assessment of the intraocular pressure is not accurate.

A special contact lens, a gonioscope, is used to examine the anterior chamber angle, to confirm that it is 'open' and to detect angle closure or other abnormal features.

Since the optic disc is the route of exit of nerve fibres from the retina to the optic nerve, and since glaucoma leads to loss of these fibres, optic disc examination is essential. The normal optic disc contains nerve fibres (the neuroretinal rim, which is pink owing to vascular perfusion), an area without nerve fibres (the optic disc cup, which is white) and blood vessels (Fig. 1). As nerve fibres are damaged and lost, the proportion of pink neuroretinal rim diminishes, the rim becomes pale and the cup enlarges (Fig. 2). This is expressed as the cup : disc ratio, which is assessed by comparing the vertical diameter of the optic disc with the vertical diameter of the cup. A cup : disc ratio of 0.6 is suggestive of glaucoma. Asymmetry between the two eyes of 0.2 is also significant (Fig. 3). An increasing cup : disc ratio is indicative of progressive disease but is difficult to detect.

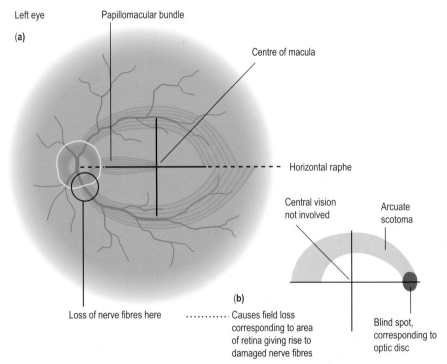

Fig. 1 **Nerve fibres entering the disc (a) and an arcuate scotoma (b).**

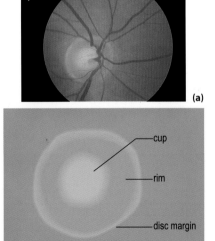

Fig. 2 **An abnormal optic disc.**

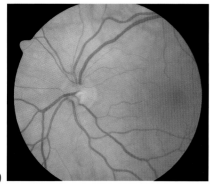

(a)

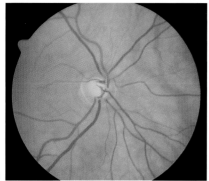

(b)

Fig. 3 **Optic disc asymmetry.**

The optic disc may be examined with the direct ophthalmoscope, but more information is obtained by stereoscopic viewing through a dilated pupil. Several instruments have been developed in an attempt to automate optic disc evaluation but are not yet in widespread clinical use. The latest are the confocal scanning laser ophthalmoscope and the scanning laser polarimeter (p. 17).

The classic visual field defect is the arcuate scotoma (Fig. 1). Confrontational testing is unlikely to reveal an abnormality. Perimeters, which are increasingly automated and computer-driven, can identify subtle loss of visual field and are therefore routinely used in the detection and follow-up of glaucoma.

Management

The only treatment thought to be effective is lowering of the intraocular pressure. In most cases this can be achieved by suppression of aqueous humour formation (drops and tablets) or increase in aqueous outflow (drops, laser trabeculoplasty and drainage surgery) (Fig. 4). Topical beta-blockers have for many years been the chief treatment for most patients, but prostaglandin derivatives are increasingly used as first line therapy (see below).

Topical aqueous humour suppression

Timolol, levobunolol, betaxolol and carteolol are all similar in efficacy. The main drawback of these agents is the potential for adverse effects through systemic absorption. In particular they may precipitate bronchospasm so that their use is contraindicated in known asthmatics and bronchitics, and may aggravate heart failure and heart block. Dorzolamide and brinzolamide are topical inhibitors of the carbonic anhydrase enzyme (important in aqueous humour production). Apraclonidine and brimonidine, which bind to alpha-adrenergic receptors, also reduce aqueous humour production. Apraclonidine can be used in the short term only.

Topical enhancement of aqueous outflow

The prostaglandin analogues latanoprost, travoprost, bimatoprost and unoprostone increase aqueous outflow through the uveoscleral route, rather than through the trabecular meshwork. They are more potent than the beta-blockers and have few systemic side-effects, so are increasingly used as first line therapy. The main unwanted effects are local: increase in iris pigmentation, increase in eyelash length and red eye. Pilocarpine, a cholinergic drug, enhances outflow through the trabecular meshwork. However, it also constricts the pupil, which may cause disabling reduction in vision in patients with cataract. In young people it impairs accommodation. It is now rarely used to treat POAG.

Other medical treatments

Adrenaline and its pro-drug dipivefrine act both to suppress aqueous production and to enhance outflow. However they are of limited efficacy and cause conjunctival irritation and inflammation. Systemic carbonic anhydrase inhibitors such as acetazolamide are very powerful, but have a range of adverse effects, including paraesthesiae, malaise, gastrointestinal upset and renal calculi, so that long-term treatment is rarely possible.

Medical treatment options for POAG are evolving rapidly. The optimal combination of drops (beta-blockers, prostaglandins, alpha-agonists, carbonic anhydrase inhibitors pilocarpine) has yet to be determined. Fixed combinations of some of these agents are available to help improve patient compliance.

Drainage surgery and other procedures

Trabeculectomy is a method of creating an opening in the anterior chamber angle for drainage. It is not always permanently successful and may aggravate cataract development, so it is usually reserved for those with failed medical treatment.

Laser surgery

The argon laser, directed at the trabecular meshwork, induces changes that lead to a lower intraocular pressure (argon laser trabeculoplasty). However the effect is not permanent and repeat treatment is not effective. Destruction of the ciliary body using laser may very effectively lower the intraocular pressure but is associated with a high rate of adverse effects.

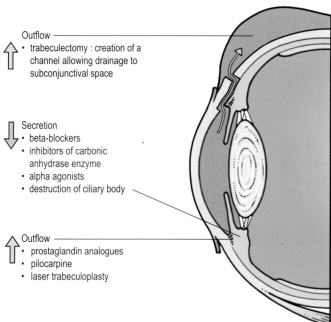

Outflow
- trabeculectomy : creation of a channel allowing drainage to subconjunctival space

Secretion
- beta-blockers
- inhibitors of carbonic anhydrase enzyme
- alpha agonists
- destruction of ciliary body

Outflow
- prostaglandin analogues
- pilocarpine
- laser trabeculoplasty

> ### Glaucoma: primary open angle
>
> - Asymptomatic: detected by optometrists and general practitioners.
> - Clinical features:
>   – optic disc cupping
>   – visual field loss
>   – open anterior chamber angle
>   – usually raised intraocular pressure.
> - Treatment:
>   – topical (prostaglandin derivatives, beta-blockers, carbonic anhydrase inhibitors, alpha-agonists)
>   – surgery when medical treatment ineffective.

Fig. 4 **Medical/surgical therapies.**

Glaucoma: angle closure and other types

Primary open angle glaucoma (POAG) accounts for about one-third of the glaucomas. Secondary glaucoma accounts for another third. Angle closure glaucoma (ACG) is usually of acute onset, presenting with pain and loss of vision, in contrast to most other glaucomas. Congenital glaucoma is rare and is often undetected until advanced. Secondary and congenital glaucoma are difficult to manage.

Acute angle closure glaucoma

Angle closure glaucoma is typically primary: the anatomy of the eye (usually hypermetropic) predisposes it to failure of aqueous humour to pass through the pupil ('pupil block') and to crowding of the anterior chamber angle, preventing aqueous access to the trabecular meshwork (Fig. 1a). The intraocular pressure rise is typically acute. Frequently a history of preceding intermittent symptoms can be elicited. The attack may resolve spontaneously, but if it becomes established, visual loss is severe and often permanent.

Clinical features
These include:

- pain, nausea, vomiting
- loss of vision
- haloes
- red eye (usually unilateral)
- cloudy cornea
- oval, non-reactive pupil
- loss of red reflex
- hypermetropia
- previous symptoms of an attack.

It is not unusual for patients with angle closure glaucoma to be admitted to hospital for investigation of vomiting, until it is realised that the eye is the cause of the symptoms. Visual loss, to 6/36 or worse, is usual, owing to corneal oedema. This is seen as a hazy cornea, which diminishes the red reflex and prevents visualisation of iris colour and structural detail. Iris ischaemia causes the pupil to be oval and non-reactive (Fig. 2).

Management
The key to correct management is making the diagnosis: no other cause of red eye leads to such pain and loss of vision, along with corneal haze and pupillary abnormality.

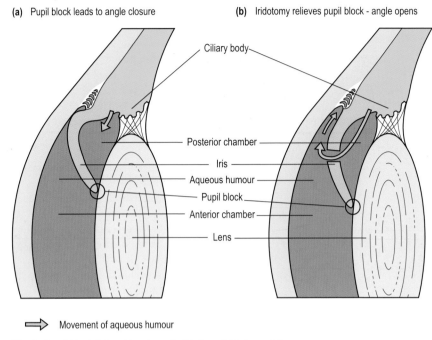

(a) Pupil block leads to angle closure   **(b)** Iridotomy relieves pupil block - angle opens

Ciliary body
Posterior chamber
Iris
Aqueous humour
Pupil block
Anterior chamber
Lens

⇒ Movement of aqueous humour

Fig. 1 **Pupil block (a) and treatment with laser iridotomy (b).**

The elevated intraocular pressure must be treated urgently, with topical and systemic aqueous suppressants (beta-blockers and acetazolamide). The pupil block can be reversed by pilocarpine. Systemic administration of analgesics and anti-emetics is welcome to the patient.

Once the acute attack has resolved, treatment to prevent recurrence and to prevent involvement of the at-risk fellow eye must be undertaken. This requires a laser iridotomy, which allows aqueous humour to pass from the posterior into the anterior chamber, by-passing the pupil (Fig. 1b).

However, it is common for the intraocular pressure to remain moderately elevated, and for the patient to require lifelong medical treatment.

A primary chronic angle closure glaucoma can also occur. This is like POAG: asymptomatic and insidious. Gonioscopy (see p. 42) is necessary to detect narrowing of the anterior chamber angle.

Secondary glaucoma
Secondary glaucoma may be open or closed angle. It may present acutely, with pain and loss of vision, or insidiously, like primary open angle glaucoma. In contrast to the latter, in which peripheral visual field loss is part of the definition, some of the secondary glaucomas feature elevated intraocular pressure alone, but with the potential to produce visual loss. Treatment is aimed first at the cause, where possible, followed by standard glaucoma treatment.

Causes
These include:

- inflammation
- pseudoexfoliation
- pigment dispersion
- aphakia
- lens abnormalities
- iris neovascularisation (rubeosis)
- steroid therapy (usually topical).

Uveitis, particularly if chronic, is likely to cause glaucoma. In children with juvenile chronic arthritis, iritis may not be acute, but associated glaucoma can be severe. Since topical steroids are the chief treatment for uveitis but may also cause a secondary glaucoma, glaucoma associated with uveitis can be especially difficult to manage.

Pseudoexfoliation and pigment dispersion are open angle glaucomas in which material (abnormal proteins in pseudoexfoliation and iris pigment in pigment dispersion) is deposited in the trabecular meshwork (Fig. 3). Onset of glaucoma is usually insidious. Both are difficult to control with medical treatment alone. Pigment dispersion most commonly affects young male myopes.

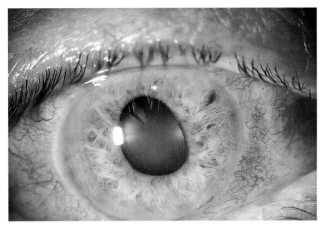

Fig. 2 **Acute angle closure glaucoma.** The eye is red and the pupil is oval. Part of the cornea is hazy.

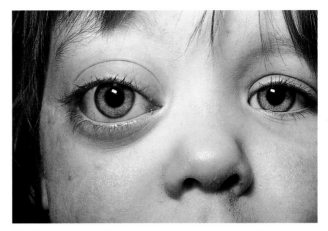

Fig. 4 **Buphthalmos.**

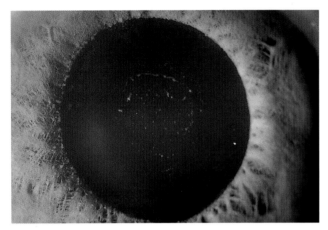

Fig. 3 **Pseudoexfoliative material on the lens.** The same material clogs up the trabecular meshwork.

The cause of aphakic glaucoma is unknown. Following surgery for paediatric cataract, it becomes increasingly prevalent with time. Management can be very difficult.

As the lens enlarges with age, it can cause narrowing of the anterior chamber angle, predisposing to angle closure glaucoma. This may be acute (pain, loss of vision) or chronic in presentation. Rarely, hypermature cataract can cause an acute inflammatory glaucoma.

Ocular ischaemia, especially retinal ischaemia (diabetic retinopathy and retinal vein occlusion), may result in anterior segment neovascularisation. New vessels grow across the surface of the iris, into the angle, which becomes closed, and within the trabecular meshwork, which becomes blocked. The resultant glaucoma is often painful and persistent.

Topical steroid use may cause secondary open angle glaucoma. Approximately 10% of the population is susceptible to an intraocular pressure rise with topical steroid use, which usually resolves on stopping treatment. However an established pressure rise can lead to irreversible glaucoma.

Management

Where possible, the primary cause should be treated: therefore inflammation is treated with steroids, retinal ischaemia with retinal photocoagulation, and lens-induced glaucoma by cataract removal. Thereafter, the sequence of medical treatment followed by surgical treatment is pursued. Surgical treatment is necessary more often than in primary open angle glaucoma, but trabeculectomy is also more likely to fail. Other surgical treatments may be needed, such as

trabeculectomy enhanced by the use of inhibitors of wound healing (5-fluorouracil and mitomycin C), tube drainage and ciliary body destruction. Tube drainage involves the insertion of a silicon tube into the anterior chamber, allowing aqueous humour to flow into a sump sutured to the eyeball. Ciliary body destruction, by laser or cryotherapy, diminishes aqueous production.

Congenital glaucoma

A variety of congenital ocular abnormalities cause glaucoma which may present at birth, in infancy or even in childhood. Primary congenital glaucoma, caused by abnormal development of the anterior chamber angle, and the secondary congenital/juvenile glaucomas are uncommon, but present major management problems.

Sturge–Weber syndrome and other phakomatoses, although present at birth, can cause a later-onset glaucoma.

The infant eyeball, unlike the adult, can enlarge enormously with elevation of intraocular pressure. This enlargement, described as **buphthalmos** ('ox eye'), is usually the presenting sign (Fig. 4). Later the cornea becomes hazy, and the eye waters. It is therefore essential that infants with watery eyes undergo a basic ocular examination.

Treatment is surgical but often fails. The prognosis is usually poor. In the case of unilateral disease, vision is rarely good, even when intraocular pressure control is satisfactory, because of amblyopia.

Glaucoma: angle closure and other types

Primary acute angle closure glaucoma
- more common in hypermetropia
- preceding history of intermittent pain, blurring and haloes
- unilateral visual loss, red eye, cloudy cornea and oval pupil
- requires urgent diagnosis and reduction of intraocular pressure – systemic acetazolamide, topical pilocarpine and beta-blockers
- fellow eye at risk – prophylactic laser iridotomy.

Secondary glaucomas
- may be open or closed angle, acute or chronic
- chief causes are uveitis, aphakia, cataract and retinal ischaemia.

Congenital glaucoma
- in infancy, the eye enlarges: buphthalmos
- visual prognosis is poor, especially in unilateral disease, owing to amblyopia.

Iritis

Iritis is the term commonly used for inflammation of the anterior uvea. However, because the anterior ciliary body is usually involved, an anatomically more correct designation is anterior uveitis or iridocyclitis. Iritis is often idiopathic (surveys vary considerably in their estimates of the proportion), but systemic associations are not uncommon. Ocular symptoms and signs are not usually indicative of a specific underlying disorder.

The cause of an idiopathic uveal inflammatory reaction is not certain, but is likely to include both genetic and environmental factors.

Anterior uveitis may be acute or chronic and can affect one or both eyes. Recurrent episodes of idiopathic acute iritis are common.

Clinical features

Symptoms
- **Pain**: an aching sensation which may be aggravated by reading.
- **Redness**.
- **Photophobia**: from reactive spasm of inflamed iris muscle.
- **Watering**.
- **Blurred vision**: secondary to inflammatory cells and flare in the anterior chamber; accommodation may be impaired.

Signs
- **Redness**. In the early stages, this may be confined to the limbal area (ciliary flush, circumcorneal injection) (Fig. 1); the eyelid conjunctiva is spared.
- **Inflammatory cells and flare**. A proteinaceous exudate in the anterior chamber is detected by slit lamp examination (the appearance is similar to the beam of a projector passing through smoke in a darkened room). If inflammation is severe, cells settle in the inferior anterior chamber angle as a hypopyon.
- **Keratic precipitates (KPs)**. KPs are clumps of inflammatory cells on the corneal endothelium, usually located on the inferior half. The size of KPs may provide a diagnostic indicator, with larger 'mutton fat' lesions typically found in association with granulomatous inflammation.
- **Miosis**. Spasm of the sphincter muscle of the pupil causes miosis. Later, focal inflammatory adhesions between the pupil margin and the lens (posterior synechiae) are caused by inflammatory mediators and are typical of iritis. They are most easily seen after pupil dilation (Fig. 2). The iris may even become atrophic or abnormally vascularised.
- **Intraocular pressure**. This can be low, high or normal.
- **Fundus**. This should be examined thoroughly, to exclude posterior uveitis and masquerade syndromes.

Figure 3 lists possible complications of recurrent or chronic iridocyclitis.

Aetiology

Patient assessment includes an attempt to detect a cause. This involves a simple systems inquiry, which may suggest appropriate investigations. Otherwise specific investigation for the most common causes is conducted only if the iritis is recurrent, persistent or bilateral.

About half of the patients with acute iridocyclitis are positive for the human leukocyte antigen (HLA) type B27, but the significance of this is not fully understood.

Ocular causes
Iritis is common in association with **herpes virus** infections of the eye and periocular structures, including herpes zoster ophthalmicus and herpes simplex keratitis. Acute glaucoma is an important complication.

Fuchs' heterochromic cyclitis is a low grade but chronic unilateral iridocyclitis characterised by heterochromia (a difference in colour between the two irides, owing to diffuse iris atrophy), fine stellate KPs across the entire endothelium and absence of posterior synechiae. Cataract and glaucoma are long-term complications. Patients usually present with 'floaters' and cataract. The iritis does not respond to treatment, but complications must be managed appropriately.

Trauma, including surgery, is a common cause of anterior segment inflammation. If the lens capsule is ruptured by trauma an intense response to exposed lens matter is usual.

Sympathetic ophthalmitis is a rare granulomatous panuveitis affecting both eyes occurring weeks to months after penetrating injury. Aggressive immunosuppressive treatment can improve an otherwise poor prognosis.

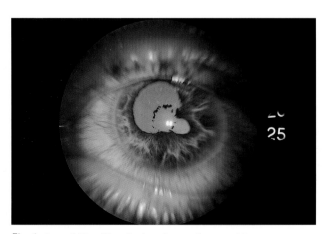

Fig. 1 **Acute iritis: ciliary flush and posterior synechiae.**

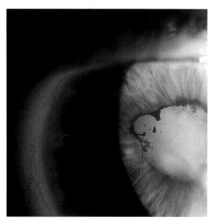

Fig. 2 **Posterior synechiae and cataract in chronic iritis.**

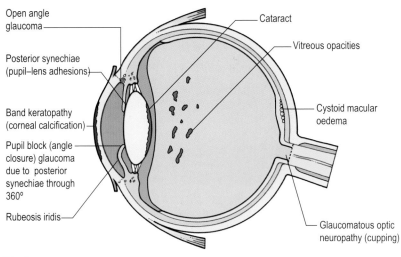

Fig. 3 **Complications of chronic iridocyclitis.**

Labels in figure:
Open angle glaucoma
Posterior synechiae (pupil–lens adhesions)
Band keratopathy (corneal calcification)
Pupil block (angle closure) glaucoma due to posterior synechiae through 360°
Rubeosis iridis
Cataract
Vitreous opacities
Cystoid macular oedema
Glaucomatous optic neuropathy (cupping)

Systemic causes

The **seronegative arthritides** are a group of related conditions in which uveitis can occur. They are frequently associated with HLA-B27 positivity.

Ankylosing spondylitis. Approximately one-third develop recurrent iritis.

Reiter's syndrome. Iritis occurs in approximately 20%.

Psoriatic arthritis (but not psoriasis alone). May be associated with iritis and conjunctivitis.

Inflammatory bowel disease (Crohn's disease, ulcerative colitis). The iridocyclitis that afflicts these patients is usually of only moderate severity. The degree of ocular inflammation may reflect that of the gastrointestinal disease.

Juvenile chronic arthritis. Chronic iridocyclitis is most strongly associated with the pauciarticular form of this disease and with a positive antinuclear antibody (ANA) test. The ocular inflammation may be insidious in onset and painless and is usually present without redness. Sight-threatening complications such as cataract, glaucoma and macular oedema are common.

Sarcoidosis. This can cause an acute, recurrent or chronic granulomatous anterior uveitis.

Behçet's disease. This is a systemic vasculitis which can cause uveitis, including acute and recurrent iridocyclitis with hypopyon, vitritis and retinal vasculitis.

Syphilis. Granulomatous or non-granulomatous acute iritis can occur with both congenital and acquired syphilis. Signs of active or inactive deep stromal corneal inflammation (interstitial keratitis) may be evident. Dilated vascular loops called roseolae are sometimes present on the surface of the iris.

Masquerade syndromes. Iritis may be simulated by a range of conditions in which uveal inflammation is not the primary pathological process. These include retinal detachment, neoplasia, bacterial endophthalmitis and the presence of an occult intraocular foreign body.

Tuberculosis. Rare.

Investigation

Systemic investigation is not usually indicated in the case of a single episode of unilateral acute anterior uveitis.

Circumstances that warrant investigation include recurrence, bilateral disease, chronicity, resistance to standard therapy and granulomatous inflammation.

Initial baseline investigations, directed by clinical suspicion, may include ESR, full blood count, a serum ACE level, syphilis serology, HLA typing and chest and sacroiliac joint X-rays.

Evidence of systemic disease should prompt referral to a physician, for further investigation and management.

Treatment

The mainstay of treatment for active iritis is the topical administration of steroids such as prednisolone, betamethasone or dexamethasone, which can be varied in concentration and frequency according to the severity of the inflammation. Drops are generally used for daytime administration, and ointment before sleep. Subconjunctival injections of steroid and mydriatic may be indicated for severe cases. Deep orbital injection of depot steroid preparations provide a higher and more stable intraocular concentration and are especially useful for posterior segment inflammation and for macular oedema. Systemic strereoids and immunosuppressants are reserved for resistant sight-threatening disease. The place of topical non-steroidal anti-inflammatory agents is poorly defined at present.

A topical mydriatic such as cyclopentolate helps to ease the discomfort and to prevent the formation of posterior synechiae.

Intraocular pressure may be elevated by the iritis itself or by topical steroid use, so should be measured regularly during active inflammation.

Iritis

- Iritis can be acute or chronic, unilateral or bilateral.
- Symptoms include pain, red eye, photophobia, lacrimation and blurred vision.
- Signs are injection, cells and flare in the anterior chamber, keratic precipitates, miosis and posterior synechiae; hypopyon occurs if inflammation is severe.
- Complications include cataract, glaucoma and macular oedema.
- A variety of systemic disorders may be associated, including ankylosing spondylitis, sarcoidosis, tuberculosis and syphilis.
- Most iritis responds to treatment with topical steroids and mydriatics.

Posterior uveitis

Posterior uveitis is inflammation of the choroid, the posterior part of the uveal tract. Inflammation of other components of the posterior part of the eye and inflammatory disorders of the pars plana of the ciliary body are also included here.

Symptoms of posterior uveitis include 'floaters' (vitreous opacities consisting of debris and inflammatory cells) and decreased vision. Pain and redness are rare.

Other causes of cells in the vitreous include neoplasia, retinal tears and HIV infection.

As with anterior uveitis, posterior uveitis can be a local disorder or part of a multisystem disease. Ophthalmoscopic features of posterior segment inflammation are shown in Figure 1 and include:

- vitritis: inflammatory cells in the vitreous
- vasculitis
- cotton wool spots
- macular oedema
- optic disc swelling
- foci of chorioretinal inflammation.

There may be a mild anterior uveitis, seen on slit lamp examination only. Investigations are summarised in Table 1.

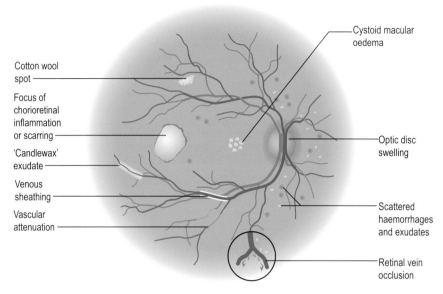

Cystoid macular oedema

Cotton wool spot

Focus of chorioretinal inflammation or scarring

'Candlewax' exudate

Venous sheathing

Vascular attenuation

Optic disc swelling

Scattered haemorrhages and exudates

Retinal vein occlusion

Fig. 1 **Ophthalmoscopic findings in posterior segment inflammation.**

Table 1 **Basic assessment in posterior segment inflammation**

Investigation	Purpose
General and ocular history	To suggest disease process and guide investigation
Fundus fluorescein angiogram	Lesions (occult vasculitis, macular oedema or ischaemia) may be disease-specific; baseline for future reference; identify cause of loss of vision
ESR	Non-specific elevation in many systemic inflammatory disorders
Complete blood count	Non-specific indicator of inflammation and general ill health
Toxoplasma serology	Negative result virtualy excludes toxoplasmosis
ACE level	Elevated in sarcoidosis
Syphilis serology	Curable disease
Chest X-ray	To detect sarcoidosis and tuberculosis

Systemic disorders

Toxoplasmosis
This is the most common cause of posterior segment inflammation in the developed world. The infective agent is a protozoan, *Toxoplasma gondii*, whose primary host is the cat. Oocysts are excreted in cat faeces and can infect humans directly or through eating the undercooked meat of infected livestock. Infection can also occur transplacentally: death in utero or major congenital abnormalities may result, though the sole clinical evidence in most cases is the incidental detection of one or more pigmented chorioretinal scars. Acquired infection tends to be subclinical but severe systemic illness can occur, particularly in immunocompromised subjects.

Reactivation of an old ocular lesion tends to occur in early adulthood, causing floaters and blurred vision. The extent of vitritis varies from a few inflammatory cells and minimal haze to dense inflammation that completely obscures the retinal view. One or more foci of activity will usually be visible in the retina as a whitish patch with moderately well defined borders and overlying vitreous inflammation, sometimes located at the edge of an old scar (Fig. 2).

The diagnosis is mainly clinical. Serological testing for toxoplasma antibodies is unhelpful, since about 50% of the general population are positive, suggesting previous exposure to the protozoa but not indicating active disease. However, a negative result in an immunocompetent patient makes a diagnosis of toxoplasma retinochoroiditis unlikely. Antibody titres generally do not rise during ocular reactivation.

Most cases of reactivation resolve spontaneously without impairment of vision so do not require treatment. Therapy, which is systemic, is indicated if vision is significantly affected or threatened, such as when a lesion is close to the macula or optic nerve. Oral steroids suppress inflammation, but concurrent antimicrobial treatment is generally used (although of unproven benefit). Appropriate antibiotics, often used in combination, include clindamycin (beware pseudomembranous colitis), sulphonamides and pyrimethamine (with folic acid).

Sarcoidosis
Sarcoidosis can affect any part of the uvea and the periocular structures. It is unusual for the fundus to be involved without some degree of anterior

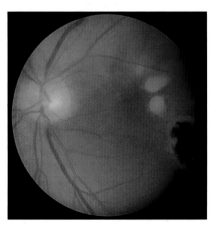

Fig. 2 **Toxoplasma chorioretinitis.**

uveitis; therefore, it tends to present with pain and redness in addition to visual symptoms. The patient, typically a young adult, may already be known to have sarcoidosis, but the first presentation can be ocular.

A systemic (especially respiratory) enquiry should be performed if sarcoidosis is suspected. Serum angiotensin-converting enzyme (ACE) and lysozyme levels and chest X-ray are useful first-line investigations.

Vitreous inflammatory cells and opacities ('snowballs'), venous sheathing and perivenous exudates ('candlewax drippings') are characteristic. Retinal and choroidal nodules may be seen. The optic disc can be swollen as a result of infiltration.

Treatment, administered in conjunction with a physician, should be directed at the systemic disease. Mild ocular inflammation may be treated with a topical steroid and a mydriatic. Periocular depot steroid injections, systemic steroids and systemic ciclosporin are reserved for severe or resistant cases in which permanent visual loss is likely.

Multisystem vasculitides
The eye may be involved in vasculitis caused by systemic lupus erythematosus, polyarteritis nodosa and Wegener's granulomatosis.

Syphilis
Syphilis is a specifically treatable condition, so it is important that it be considered in the differential diagnosis of any posterior uveitis with non-specific signs. Iridocyclitis, vitritis, occlusive vasculitis and chorioretinitis of variable pattern can all occur. Treatment is with penicillin or erythromycin.

Congenital syphilitic chorioretinitis results in a pigmentary retinopathy in a 'salt-and-pepper' pattern.

Toxocariasis
Toxocariasis is caused by a roundworm, which is passed on to young children from dogs. Ocular disease usually presents with vitritis and a solitary choroidal granuloma. There may be leukocoria (Table 2, p. 50). The visual prognosis is poor.

Tuberculosis
Chronic granulomatous anterior uveitis is the typical ocular manifestation of tuberculosis. Multiple foci of chorioretinitis as part of systemic military disease may occur. Treatment is of the underlying disease.

Cytomegalovirus retinitis
This is seen almost exclusively in immunocompromised patients, particularly those with acquired immune deficiency syndrome (AIDS). Presentation is with painless visual loss, often bilateral. White areas of necrotic retinal exudate mixed with flame haemorrhages are said to resemble a pizza. There is minimal anterior chamber or vitreous activity. Treatment options include systemic or intravitreal ganciclovir, oral valganciclovir, intravenous foscarnet and cidofovir. Resolution leaves a highly atrophic retina which is prone to detach.

Candidiasis
Candida endophthalmitis is an opportunistic infection that tends to be confined to patients with predisposing factors, including immunosuppression, indwelling intravenous catheters and intravenous drug abuse. A multifocal chorioretinitis and vitritis is usual. Systemic antifungal agents are necessary.

Behçet's disease
Ocular features include anterior uveitis, typically with a hypopyon, and an occlusive vasculitis. Venous occlusion and macular oedema are typical.

Vogt–Koyanagi–Harada (VKH) syndrome
Neurological and cutaneous manifestations are found in this multisystem granulomatous condition affecting dark-skinned individuals. Anterior and posterior uveitis with localised exudative retinal detachment are amongst the diagnostic features.

Miscellaneous localised disorders
Most of these conditions are very rare. Fundus fluorescein angiography may help with diagnosis.

Ocular histoplasmosis syndrome
Rare in the UK but relatively common in the southern USA and elsewhere, this condition is thought to be associated with infection by the fungus *Histoplasma capsulatum*. Discrete atrophic lesions, a predisposition to choroidal neovascularisation and an absence of inflammatory signs are the hallmarks.

Sympathetic ophthalmitis
This is a bilateral granulomatous panuveitis which very occasionally follows penetrating trauma to one or both eyes. Aggressive anti-inflammatory treatment is urgently indicated.

Acute posterior multifocal placoid pigment epitheliopathy (AMPPE)
AMPPE presents in young adults shortly after a viral illness, with blurred vision owing to patchy exudative retinal detachment. Spontaneous resolution to normal occurs in a few weeks.

Acute retinal necrosis
It is thought that herpes virus infection may cause this condition, in which retinal necrosis advances from the periphery towards the centre.

Others
Other rare ocular inflammations, the causes of which are unknown, include birdshot retinochoroidopathy, serpiginous choroidopathy, punctate inner choroidopathy and multiple evanescent white dot syndrome.

Pars planitis
Pars planitis, which typically affects teenagers and young adults, presents with floaters and blurred vision in one or both eyes. There are inflammatory cells and opacities in the anterior vitreous. There may also be cystoid macular oedema, the chief cause of visual loss. In the area of the anterior retina and pars plana, which is difficult to visualise, there will be the pathognomonic feature of 'snowbanking' (exudation). Cataract is common. The cause is unknown.

Treatment is required only if vision is significantly decreased, to 6/12 or worse. First-line treatment is an intensive course of a topical steroid. Orbital injection and systemic steroids are occasionally necessary.

Posterior uveitis

- Symptoms of posterior segment inflammation are floaters and blurred vision; there is usually no pain or redness.
- Posterior uveitis can be a feature of systemic disease.
- Baseline investigations: fundus fluorescein angiogram, ESR, CBC, ACE level, serology for toxoplasma and syphilis, chest X-ray.
- Pars planitis is an inflammation of the ciliary body that causes vitreous floaters, macular oedema and cataract. Treat with topical, periocular, or systemic steroids.
- A number of rare inflammatory disorders localised to the eye can occur.

The lens

The most frequently seen disorder of the lens is loss of clarity, termed cataract, which causes a variety of symptoms. Displacement of the lens, ectopia lentis, is rare.

Cataract

Cataract is very common. Almost everybody over the age of 70 has some degree of lenticular opacity, although many remain asymptomatic and relatively few require surgery.

Congenital and infantile cataract differ morphologically and aetiologically from age-related opacity.

Aetiology

The majority of cataract encountered in clinical practice is associated with 'normal' age-related degenerative change (**senile cataract**).

The pathogenesis has yet to be determined, but ultraviolet light has been implicated. Cataract presenting in a young or early middle-aged person with no apparent cause should prompt further investigation (Table 1).

Congenital or infantile cataract is frequently an isolated finding. About a third are inherited in an autosomal dominant fashion. Another third are caused by birth trauma or maternal infection during pregnancy, particularly rubella and toxoplasmosis. These infections typically result in a variety of additional systemic abnormalities. Galactosaemia is the most common metabolic cause of congenital or infantile cataract. Wilson's disease, Lowe's syndrome and Fabry's disease are rare causes.

Morphology

Morphologic variants typical of particular aetiologies are seen, such as posterior subcapsular opacity in steroid-related cataract and the 'oil-drop' appearance of galactosaemia. The appearance of congenital cataract varies but tends to involve the nucleus, the earliest part of the lens to develop in utero.

Senile cataract takes the form of one or a combination of (Fig. 1):

- nuclear sclerosis: gradually deepening diffuse brunescence
- subcapsular: shallow opacification just beneath the capsule, more commonly posterior than anterior
- cortical: discrete spoke-like opacities of the cortex.

Clinical assessment

Disturbance of vision is the usual presenting symptom. This may be

Table 1 **Pre-senile cataract – causes**
Systemic disorders causing cataract:
■ diabetes mellitus
■ corticosteroid therapy
■ atopy
■ galactosaemia
■ hypocalcaemia
■ dystrophia myotonica
Ocular factors causing cataract:
■ blunt or perforating trauma
■ high myopia
■ recurrent uveitis
■ topical steroid use
■ ionising irradiation
■ excessive ultraviolet light exposure
■ infrared irradiation.

Table 2 **Causes of leukocoria**
Cataract
Toxocara granuloma
Retinoblastoma
Advanced retinopathy of prematurity
Retinal dysplasias
Vitreous maldevelopment (persistent hyperplastic primary vitreous)
Corneal opacity
Coat's disease

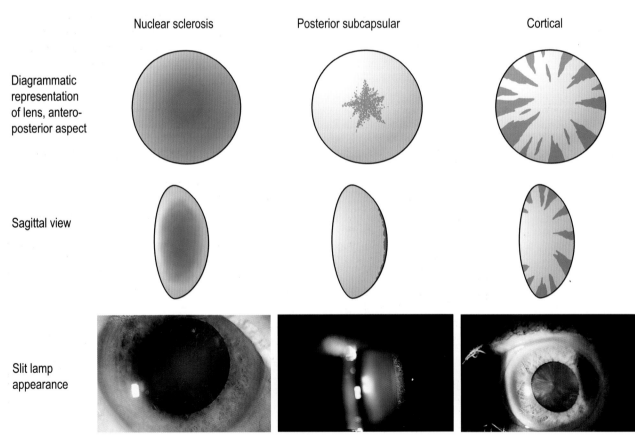

Fig. 1 **Morphological variants of senile cataract.**

gradual loss of clarity with dimness of vision, progressive myopia caused by increasing density of the nucleus (nuclear sclerosis), glare or monocular diplopia. Symptoms may vary with changes in ambient illumination, as the pupil constricts and dilates. If cataract is predominantly uniocular, it may go unnoticed until the other eye becomes affected.

Infants and children do not complain of visual loss. Cataract may be detected at a routine development check-up, or in family photographs when a white pupil (leukocoria; Table 2) becomes obvious.

History and examination are directed at determining the level of visual impairment and at detecting a cause. Snellen visual acuity is always measured but correlates poorly with functional impairment. Since the prognosis for visual recovery after surgery depends especially on retinal health, dilated fundal examination is mandatory. If the retina cannot be seen, field of vision testing using a light or hand-waving, pupil testing for RAPD (p. 15) and ultrasonic examination (to exclude retinal detachment or tumour) should be performed.

A cataract can be detected by examination of the red reflex after pupil dilation, using the direct ophthalmoscope (Fig. 1).

Consideration should also be given to general health, particularly when deciding on the mode of anaesthesia: general, regional block or topical.

In children, cataract must be differentiated from the other causes of leukocoria (Table 2). Examination under general anaesthesia, ultrasound and electrophysiology may be required. A paediatrician will be able to help to determine the aetiology.

Cataract surgery

Increasingly sophisticated techniques of cataract removal and refinements in artificial lens technology have revolutionised the management of cataract. Surgery is safe, quick and cost-effective and is being performed at an increasingly early stage in cataract development.

However, complications occur in a small minority and can be devastating. If the retina cannot be adequately examined preoperatively, the prognosis is guarded until the post-operative period.

Cataract in children poses a particular management problem, since simple removal of the opacity does not restore vision: principal difficulties are correction of the aphakia and management of amblyopia. The eye may still be growing, so that lens implantation is controversial. Amblyopia is likely to limit visual improvement, especially in unilateral cataract.

Indications for surgery

Surgery to improve visual function depends on the degree of impairment and the visual needs of the individual.

Other indications include diabetic retinopathy, when cataract prevents adequate retinal examination or laser treatment, and lens-induced glaucoma or uveitis.

Principles of surgery

Surgery is described elsewhere (see pg. 92). Principal considerations include:

- choice of anaesthesia
- incision: via cornea or anterior sclera
- technique of cataract removal
- correction of aphakia: by intraocular lens implantation, contact lens or aphakic spectacles.

Prognosis

Eighty per cent of eyes achieve 6/12 vision or better following surgery. Failure to improve is usually due to pre-existing disease. Posterior capsule opacification after successful surgery will reduce vision but can be treated by laser capsulotomy.

Ectopia lentis (Table 3)

Ectopia lentis is the partial or complete dislocation of the lens from its physiological position (Fig. 2). It may be associated with glaucoma.

Contact lenses may need to be worn to overcome the refractive consequence of ectopia lentis. In some cases, surgical removal of the dislocated lens may be necessary. Paradoxically the optical effects of partial dislocation are more disabling than complete dislocation.

Table 3 **Ectopia lentis – causes**	
Acquired causes:	**Hereditary causes:**
■ trauma	■ Marfan's syndrome (upward dislocation)
■ hypermature cataractous lens	■ Homocystinuria
■ anterior intraocular tumour	■ Weill-Marchesani syndrome
■ syphilis	

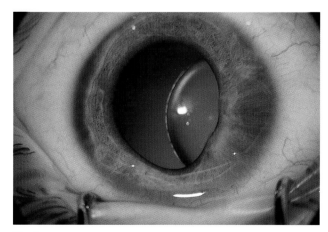

Fig. 2 **A dislocated lens.**

The lens

Cataract
- symptoms: decreased vision, glare, monocular diplopia, change in refraction
- systemic associations include diabetes, corticosteroid therapy, metabolic disorders
- clinical assessment: degree of functional impairment; presence of other ocular or systemic pathology
- prognosis: excellent if no other ocular disease; surgical complication rate is low
- failure to improve: pre-existing disease, such as amblyopia, macular degeneration, retinal vein occlusion, glaucoma.

Congenital cataract
- exclude other causes of leukocoria
- systemic assessment with paediatrician
- poorer prognosis than adult cataract, owing to amblyopia.

Ectopia lentis
- trauma, hypermature cataract, Marfan's syndrome
- complications: refractive problems, secondary glaucoma
- lens removal may be necessary.

Ocular fundus: diabetic retinopathy

Diabetes mellitus can affect the visual system directly and indirectly in a variety of ways. The complication usually associated with diabetes is retinopathy, but extraocular muscle palsy, stroke, retinal vascular occlusions and cataract are all relatively common in diabetics. Many of the complications of retinopathy can be modified by early detection and treatment.

Epidemiology

Twenty years after diagnosis, virtually all Type I (early onset, usually insulin-dependent) diabetics and approximately 60% of Type II (later onset, usually non-insulin dependent) diabetics will have retinopathy detectable on examination, though not all of these will have symptoms. After 30 years, 30% of Type I and 3% of Type II diabetics will have developed proliferative disease.

Aetiopathogenesis

Hyperglycaemia is believed to be the primary cause of the microvascular complications of diabetes, including the retinopathy. Glycosylation of tissue proteins may play a major role. The clinical manifestations can by explained by the twin processes of small vessel occlusion and increased permeability (loss of the blood-retinal barrier) (Fig. 1). Changes in the vessel wall and loss of supporting pericytes occur. Increased red cell and platelet stickiness and reduced oxygen transport also contribute to an ischaemic tendency. Proliferation of new vessels (neovascularisation) occurs in response to vasogenic factors released by ischaemic retina.

Clinical presentation

Retinopathy is frequently detected during routine screening of a known diabetic, before the onset of symptoms. Screening is now a requirement of healthcare providers.

Visual loss is usually caused by maculopathy or vitreous haemorrhage. Visual loss in maculopathy may be slight at first, but without treatment is gradually progressive. Vitreous haemorrhage, in contrast, is often acute and dense, with severe loss of vision. Small haemorrhages suspended within the vitreous gel cause the appearance of a net curtain or blot in the vision.

Clinical features

Microaneurysms (focal capillary dilatations) and dot haemorrhages are

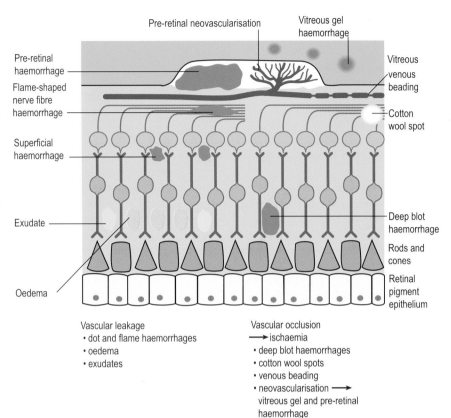

Fig. 1 **Diagrammatic representation of the consequences of vascular leakage and occlusion, showing the retina in cross-section.**

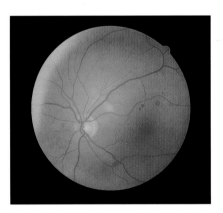

Fig. 2 **Background diabetic retinopathy** (left eye).

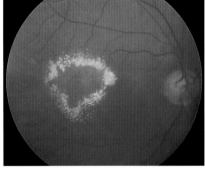

Fig. 3 **Circinate pattern of exudates at the macula** (right eye).

very similar in appearance (Fig. 2). Blot haemorrhages are darker and larger. Exudates (Figs 2 & 3), discrete yellow deposits of protein-rich material, should be differentiated from whiter, fluffy cotton wool spots (Fig. 4). Exudates occur due to leakage whereas cotton wool spots are swollen axons. Large numbers of cotton wool spots indicate significant ischaemia (Fig. 4). Retinal oedema is difficult to detect, but since oedematous retina loses its transparency, involved retina is dull and loses its normal sheen. At the centre of the macula, the oedema is cystoid in appearance.

Venous changes are subtle but important to detect. Loops, doubling and beading occur (Fig. 4). Severity is graded according to the number of quadrants of affected retina.

Neovascularisation (Fig. 5) may remain within the retina (intraretinal microvascular anomalies, or IRMAs) or may project forwards into the vitreous. New vessels are fragile, so bleed easily, and are accompanied by a fibrotic element. This contractile structure can lead to tractional retinal detachment.

Classification

The changes of diabetic retinopathy have traditionally been divided into

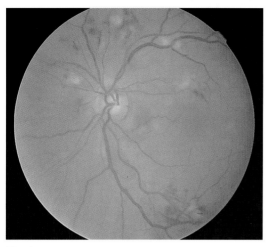

Fig. 4 **Pre-proliferative retinopathy** (left eye). Note cotton wool spots and venous beading.

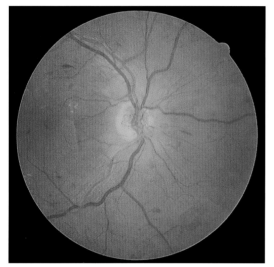

Fig. 5 **Proliferative retinopathy** (right eye). Note new vessels at the disc and IRMA inferonasally.

background, pre-proliferative and proliferative grades (Table 1). The clinical features of each represent the relative contributions of the leakage (background) and occlusive (proliferation) mechanisms. Thus background changes consist of microaneurysms, dot and blot haemorrhages, exudates and oedema. In preproliferative retinopathy there are marked venous changes, cotton wool spots and IRMAs. There is a substantial likelihood of progression to pre-retinal neovascularisation.

Neovascularisation occurs at the optic disc or elsewhere, usually along the temporal vascular arcades. In maculopathy, changes similar to background retinopathy are present. If advanced diabetic eye disease occurs, treatment has failed and the eye is blind. There may be neovascularisation on the iris (rubeosis, leading to a severe glaucoma), persistent vitreous haemorrhage and tractional retinal detachment.

Differential diagnosis

Retinal vein occlusions and hypertensive retinopathy may give a fundus appearance similar to diabetic retinopathy.

Management

Screening and prevention

Treatment of established retinopathy may fail to prevent sight loss, so prevention of sight-threatening retinopathy is the goal (Table 2). Hence, the development of screening procedures is essential. All diabetics should undergo fundus examination at least once a year. The best method of screening has yet to be determined. Techniques include direct ophthalmoscopy by an optometrist, general practitioner or diabetes physician, and fundus photography, with examination of photographs by a specialist or trained technician.

Effective control of hyperglycaemia can retard both the onset of retinopathy and its progression, and it is important to emphasise this to the patient. As with other diabetic complications, hypertension has a synergistic effect so that optimal control is essential. Smoking should be stopped.

Several pharmacological agents, such as protein kinase C inhibitors, may have the potential to modify the development of diabetic retinopathy and are currently under investigation.

Since sight loss is caused by maculopathy and proliferative retinopathy, patients should be referred for ophthalmological assessment if maculopathy or preproliferative or proliferative retinopathy is suspected.

Specialist ophthalmic management

Application of an ocular laser is the chief treatment. In areas of macular oedema, the laser reduces focal leakage and improves reabsorption of retinal oedema. Fundus fluorescein angiography can help to identify treatable lesions. Reversing proliferative retinopathy requires lasering of ischaemic areas, to reduce the neovascular stimulus. Clearly, this causes loss of potentially useful retina, so application has to be titrated against the response to laser treatment. The treatment of preproliferative retinopathy is controversial, but severe changes warrant prophylactic laser application.

The presence of vitreous haemorrhage represents screening or treatment failure. Although haemorrhage may resorb spontaneously, it may persist, preventing observation and laser treatment. Persistent haemorrhage can be removed by a vitrectomy procedure. Tractional retinal detachment is difficult to treat and the visual outcome is usually poor.

Table 1 **Classification of diabetic retinopathy**	
Grade of retinopathy	**Features**
Background	Microaneurysms
	Dot and blot haemorrhages
	Exudates
Preproliferative	Cotton wool spots
	Venous beading, loops and doubling
Proliferative	New vessels at the disc (NVD)
	New vessels elsewhere (NVE)
Maculopathy	Microaneurysms, haemorrhages, exudates, oedema at the macula
Advanced disease	Iris rubeosis, persistent vitreous haemorrhage, retinal detachment

Table 2 **Risk of severe visual loss* after two years: the effect of panretinal laser photocoagulation**		
	Untreated	**Treated**
New vessels at the disc plus vitreous haemorrhage	40%	20%
Prominent new vessels elsewhere plus vitreous haemorrhage	30%	7%
New vessels elsewhere, no vitreous haemorrhage	7%	7%
*Severe visual loss = worse than 6/240		

Ocular fundus: diabetic retinopathy

■ More common and more aggressive in Type I diabetics.

■ Small vessel disease: occlusion and increased permeability.

■ Symptoms are usually due to maculopathy or vitreous haemorrhage.

■ Clinical features include microaneurysms, exudates, haemorrhages (dot, blot, flame), cotton wool spots, oedema, venous beading, neovascularisation.

■ Treatments: macular laser for maculopathy, panretinal laser for neovascularisation, vitrectomy for persistent vitreous haemorrhage.

Ocular fundus: retinal vascular occlusions

Retinal venous and arterial occlusions are among the more common serious ophthalmic conditions presenting acutely. They should always be considered in the differential diagnosis of a patient with sudden painless loss of vision (Table 1). Since retinal vascular occlusion is usually a manifestation of a systemic disease, patient evaluation should always include a systemic assessment. In determining the cause, consider Virchow's triad, of 'outside the wall', 'in the wall' and 'in the lumen' (Fig. 1).

Retinal vein occlusion

Venous occlusions can affect the central retinal vein or a tributary – a 'branch' retinal vein occlusion.

Aetiopathogenesis

Thrombosis occurs within the lumen of the vessel. In branch occlusions, this is frequently seen at an arteriovenous crossing point. Abnormalities of blood constituents may promote thrombus formation.

Clinical presentation

Patients are typically middle-aged or elderly. Sudden painless loss of central vision occurs when the involved segment of retina includes the macula, as is the case with central and some branch occlusions. The severity of the initial fall in visual acuity varies considerably from case to case, commonly ranging from 6/9 to 'hand movements'. There may be a relative afferent pupillary defect. On fundoscopy flame, dot and blot haemorrhages, cotton wool spots, a swollen optic disc and macular oedema may be seen (Fig. 2).

Table 1 **Chief causes of sudden painless monocular loss of vision**	
■ Retinal vein occlusion	■ Macular haemorrhage (especially 'wet' macular degeneration)
■ Retinal artery occlusion	■ Optic neuritis
■ Anterior ischaemic optic neuropathy	■ Retinal detachment
■ Vitreous haemorrhage	

In a branch vein occlusion, changes are confined to the area of retina drained by the blocked vessel.

The condition is usually unilateral. The two major complications are macular oedema and neovascularisation of the iris and retina. Iris neovascularisation (rubeosis) can lead to a severe, painful glaucoma which is difficult to control.

Patient assessment

Common systemic associations include hypertension and diabetes. Rarely, blood dyscrasias or vasculitis may be the cause. The major ocular association is elevated intraocular pressure.

The diagnosis is clinical. Investigations are directed primarily at excluding treatable associations.

Treatment

Treatment is of the disease and of any systemic association.

- Macular oedema – laser treatment to reduce oedema and improve vision may be successful in branch retinal vein occlusion.
- Neovascularisation – as with proliferative diabetic retinopathy, laser of ischaemic areas can reverse neovascularisation. The case for prophylactic laser after vein occlusion but before the development of neovascularisation is not yet proven.
- Neovascular glaucoma – a variety of treatments, including laser and surgery, are used, but the outcome is usually poor. A painful blind eye may need to be removed.

Retinal artery occlusion

Arterial occlusions typically lead to more severe visual loss than venous occlusions. As with venous disease, arterial occlusion can involve the central artery itself or one of its branches.

Aetiopathogenesis

The commonest cause of arterial occlusion is embolisation, the embolus originating most frequently from a source in a

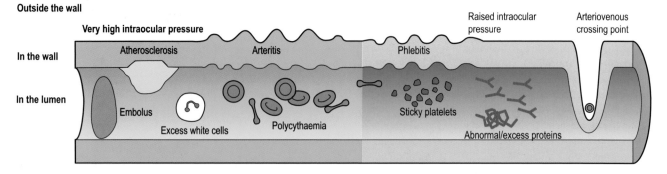

Fig. 1 **Causes of retinal vascular occlusion.**

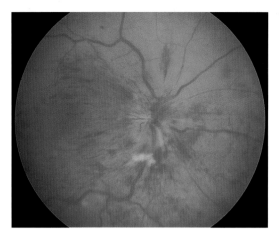

Fig. 2 **Central retinal vein occlusion (right eye).**

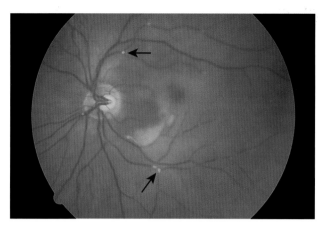

Fig. 4 **Retinal emboli.** Partially macular oedema and a cherry-red spot are also shown.

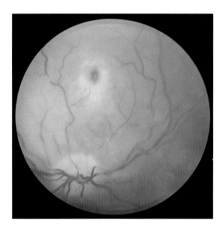

Fig. 3 **Cherry-red spot in central retinal artery occlusion.**

carotid artery and consisting of cholesterol, calcific plaques or fibrinoplatelet material. Emboli may pass through the retinal vascular system, causing transient rather than permanent visual loss. A stationary embolus, however, causes retinal failure in the territory beyond the point of obstruction. Inflammation within the vessel wall, arteritis, may also cause occlusion.

Clinical presentation
A branch retinal arteriolar occlusion may not give symptoms if the area affected is away from the macula. Central artery occlusions usually present with the sudden onset of severe monocular loss of vision, often to 'counting fingers' or worse. The patient may report having experienced similar but transient episodes previously (amaurosis fugax).

A marked relative afferent pupillary defect is usually present in central occlusions and frequently in branch artery occlusions.

In the first few weeks following the acute event, the affected retinal arterioles may be seen to be thinned, with segmentation of the columns of blood. Unlike ischaemic optic neuropathy, the optic disc is not usually pale or swollen. The oedematous retina is devoid of its usual glistening appearance and may appear whitish and opaque. At the centre of the macula, where the thinner retina allows greater visibility of the unaffected highly vascular choroid, a 'cherry-red spot' is usual (Fig. 3). One or two cotton wool spots are a common finding. Similar signs are evident in both branch and central retinal artery occlusions but in the branch form the changes are confined to the portion of the retina supplied by that vessel. Emboli may be seen within the arterioles (Fig. 4).

After approximately six weeks the cherry-red spot recedes. Optic disc pallor becomes evident due to loss of the axons of the retinal ganglion cells.

Unlike other ischaemic retinal diseases, neovascularisation is uncommon.

Patient assessment
Patients often have systemic conditions associated with microvascular disease, particularly hypertension, diabetes

mellitus, ischaemic heart disease and peripheral vascular disease, and a history of cigarette smoking. Giant cell arteritis, although usually causing ischaemic optic neuropathy rather than embolic retinal artery occlusion, should always be considered. Key features are pain and tenderness along the superficial temporal artery and elevated erythrocyte sedimentation rate and C-reactive protein. Other investigations may be performed to detect occult cardiovascular disease and potential sources of embolisation. In particular, carotid ultrasound ('Duplex') scanning may show significant stenosis.

Treatment
There is no specific treatment which reliably restores vision, but urgent referral to confirm the diagnosis is necessary, especially if a diagnosis of giant cell arteritis, which is treatable, is not to be missed (Table 1). Regular prophylactic aspirin is prescribed, if not contraindicated, since it is likely to have a protective effect against arterial occlusion in the other eye and against stroke. In some patients with carotid stenosis, carotid endarterectomy may be indicated to reduce the risk of further embolic episodes.

Occular fundus: retinal vascular occlusions

■ Retinal vascular occlusions are:
  – usually unilateral
  – associated with systemic disease.

■ Key features of retinal vein occlusion:
  – tortuous dilated veins
  – flame haemorrhages localised to area drained by affected vein.

■ Key features of retinal artery occlusion:
  – history of amaurosis fugax
  – retinal pallor, cherry-red spot
  – narrow truncated arteries
  – embolus.

Ocular fundus: other retinal vascular disorders

Hypertensive retinopathy

Various classification systems have been proposed to grade the ophthalmoscopic findings in hypertension. The retinal changes mirror the systemic circulation, and their severity correlates well with the development of the systemic complications of hypertension and with survival.

Retinal vascular changes in hypertension comprise:

- the vasospastic reaction to an acute pressure rise (the true hypertensive response)
- the arteriolosclerotic response to chronic elevation.

Clinical features

Generalised arteriolar narrowing

Arteriolosclerosis occurs through medial hyperplasia and fibrosis resulting from chronically elevated pressure. Slowly progressive arteriolosclerosis is a feature of normal ageing. On ophthalmoscopy, there is broadening of the arteriolar light reflex ('burnished copper', 'polished silver') and venous nipping at arteriovenous crossing points.

Focal arteriolar narrowing

A vasospastic effect occurring in response to an acute pressure rise.

Flame haemorrhages

These are located in the nerve fibre layer (Fig. 1) and result from capillary damage. Dot and blot haemorrhages can also develop.

Cotton wool spots

Small feathery white spots consisting of swollen axonal endings (Fig. 1) are caused by focal ischaemia.

Exudates

Well-defined yellow-white intraretinal collections of lipid are derived from vascular leakage and vary in size. At the macula, a 'star' may develop, consisting of exudates arranged in a bicycle spoke-like pattern radiating from its centre (Fig. 2).

Optic disc swelling

This is thought to be caused by local ischaemia. Rarely there is raised intracranial pressure (true papilloedema).

Arteriolar macroaneurysms

These localised arteriolar dilations (Fig. 3) are strongly associated with hypertension and arteriolosclerosis. Macroaneurysms are prone to leak blood and serous fluids. Symptomatic lesions at the macula are ablated using laser.

Microaneurysms

These are similar to the lesions occurring in diabetic retinopathy and are well-defined red dots.

These features are summarised in Table 1.

Malignant hypertension

Malignant hypertension is the clinical syndrome of an accelerated rise in blood pressure. Untreated, mortality at 1 year is 90%. In the retina, it is characterised by Grade 4 hypertensive changes (Table 1).

Retinopathy of prematurity (ROP)

This fibrovascular retinal proliferative disorder occurs in premature and low birth weight babies. Its development is associated with high inhaled oxygen concentration during the neonatal period. Other less well-defined risk factors, such as maternal smoking, neonatal sepsis and blood transfusion, have been implicated.

Normal retinal vascularisation is not complete until full-term gestation. It is thought that in the premature baby, normal retinal vascularisation ceases, perhaps because of adequate oxygenation from inspired air, then either continues normally (resolved ROP) or proceeds in an abnormal manner, vessels growing forwards into the vitreous cavity. These vessels may bleed. The associated fibrous component can contract, detaching the retina.

Table 1	Retinal changes in hypertension and arteriolosclerosis
Grade	**Features**
	Hypertension
1	Generalised arteriolar narrowing
2	More marked generalised narrowing with irregular points of focal constriction
3	Generalised and focal narrowing plus cotton wool spots, retinal haemorrhages, hard exudates
4	As grade 3 but with swelling of the optic disc
	Arteriolosclerosis
1	Decreased venular visibility at arteriovenous crossing points, slight broadening of the arteriolar light reflex
2	Deflection of the venule at arteriovenous crossing points
3	'Copper wire' arterioles, marked venular narrowing and deflection at crossing points
4	'Silver wire' arterioles, extreme crossing changes

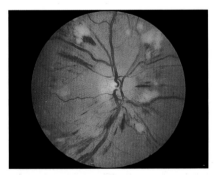

Fig. 1 **Flame haemorrhages and cotton wool spots in hypertensive retinopathy.**

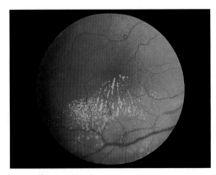

Fig. 2 **Macular exudates ('star') in hypertensive retinopathy.**

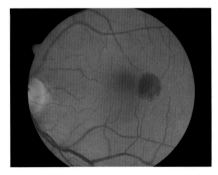

Fig. 3 **Haemorrhage from a macroaneurysm.**

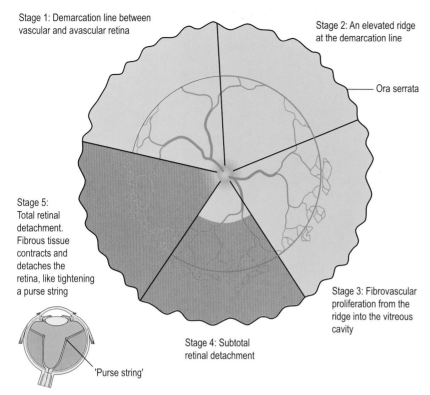

Stage 1: Demarcation line between vascular and avascular retina

Stage 2: An elevated ridge at the demarcation line

Ora serrata

Stage 5: Total retinal detachment. Fibrous tissue contracts and detaches the retina, like tightening a purse string

'Purse string'

Stage 3: Fibrovascular proliferation from the ridge into the vitreous cavity

Stage 4: Subtotal retinal detachment

Fig. 4 **The stages of ROP.**

Clinical features

Active ROP may progress through five stages of increasing severity (Fig. 4), culminating in total retinal detachment. Spontaneous regression of the earlier stages occurs without intervention in a majority, but sequelae may still cause sight loss. The more anterior the limit of vascularised retina at the time of the development of active ROP (the 'zone' of the ROP), the better the prognosis.

Other changes that have poor prognostic significance are also recognised ('plus' disease): dilated veins and tortuous arteries at the posterior pole, vitreous haemorrhage and iris vascularisation.

Premature babies are also susceptible to strabismus and myopia, and to intracranial haemorrhage causing cortical blindness.

Screening

Screening is recommended for babies born at or less than 31 weeks' gestational age and for those weighing less than 1500 g at birth. Dilated fundal examination is carried out regularly from 6 or 7 weeks after birth until the nasal retina is fully vascularised. A very premature subgroup are screened more intensively.

Treatment

Treatment is indicated for 'threshold' disease (defined as extensive stage 3 changes). This is the severity of disease that is likely to progress to visual loss and at which the benefits of treatment outweigh the risks. The avascular area is ablated using either cryotherapy or laser to induce regression of abnormally growing new vessels. These babies often have other medical problems that make treatment hazardous. Surgery for retinal detachment has had only very limited success.

Sickle-cell retinopathy

Mutant haemoglobin, such as sickle haemoglobin S, causes red blood cells to behave abnormally, in particular making them less flexible and unable to pass freely through small blood vessels. Hypoxia exacerbates this tendency. Combinations of abnormal haemoglobins occur: the most common, and the least severe, is haemoglobin S combined with normal haemoglobin A (sickle trait). Haemoglobin S is common in blacks but extremely rare in whites.

Sickle-cell retinopathy is caused by the impaction of deformed red cells in the retinal vasculature, leading to occlusion and ischaemia. Paradoxically, sickle cell disease (pure haemoglobin S) does not cause the most severe retinopathy.

Clinical features

Systemic manifestations include anaemia and sickle crises.
The eye shows two types of change:

- **Proliferative retinopathy**. Peripheral proliferative changes develop after vascular occlusion and arteriovenous anastomosis. The new vessels resemble a fan ('sea-fan' neovascularisation). Vitreous haemorrhage may occur. Progressive contraction of fibrovascular tissue may lead to tractional retinal detachment or to the formation of retinal tears.
- **Non-proliferative retinopathy**. Black 'sunburst' scars and 'salmon-patch' retinal haemorrhages are probably a result of infarction. Venous tortuosity is common. Retinal artery or vein occlusion may occur.

Management

Patients with sickle disease should be screened for retinopathy at regular intervals and observed more frequently if signs develop. Laser photocoagulation is performed for neovascularisation.

Ocular fundus: other retinal vascular disorders

- Hypertensive retinopathy involves an arteriolosclerotic and a vasospastic response.
- Retinopathy of prematurity:
  - can resolve naturally or progress through five stages
  - premature and low birth weight babies should be screened
  - 'threshold' ROP (extensive stage 3) is treated with laser or cryotherapy to the avascular area
  - high incidence of myopia and strabismus.
- Threshold (ROP) disease (extensive stage 3) is treated with laser or cryotherapy to the avascular area.
- Sickle-cell retinopathy involves proliferative ('sea-fan' neovascularisation) and non-proliferative ('black sunbursts', 'salmon-patch' haemorrhages, venous tortuosity, vascular occlusion) changes. The former are treated with laser photocoagulation.

Ocular fundus: macular disease I

Macular degeneration

Age-related macular degeneration (AMD or ARMD) is the most common reason for blind registration in the western world. It is a disorder associated with increasing age and is typically bilateral. Despite causing 'blindness', it does in fact result in loss of central vision only. Thus peripheral vision, important for navigation, is retained. For this reason, sufferers are generally able to maintain an independent lifestyle.

Classification

Macular degeneration can be considered 'dry', in cases where there is slowly progressive deterioration in visual function, and 'wet' when growth of new, abnormally located blood vessels (a choroidal neovascular membrane, or CNVM) underneath the retina causes sudden loss of vision, by leakage of fluid or by haemorrhage.

Pathology (Fig. 1)

The principal feature is the presence of drusen, deposited between the retinal pigment epithelium (RPE) and the underlying Bruch's membrane. There is atrophy of retinal pigment epithelial cells and degenerative change in photoreceptor outer segments. These changes are concentrated at the macula; hence the term macular degeneration.

In the 'wet' form of the disease a vascular membrane may grow from the choroidal layer towards the retina.

Clinical features

Usually, there is progressive, gradual loss of central vision, leading to difficulty with reading and with recognising distant objects. Peripheral

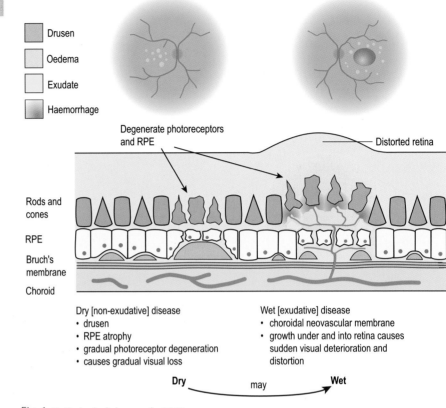

Fig. 1 **Pathological changes in AMD.**

vision is retained, so patients are able to navigate satisfactorily. In the 'wet' form, the visual disturbance is often sudden, causing profound central visual loss or, if retinal function is maintained, distortion of straight lines: doorways and reading print seem to bend (Fig. 2). If the process occurs eccentric to the fovea, these symptoms may be appreciated as off-centre. Pupil reactions are usually normal.

Drusen, small discrete yellowish deposits (Fig. 3), are commonly seen at the macula after the age of 45 years, but they are usually asymptomatic. With increasing age, their size and number increase. The macula becomes mottled due to atrophic pallor and reactive hyperpigmentation (Fig. 3). Even at this advanced stage, clinical appearances correlate poorly with measured visual acuity.

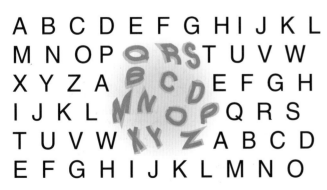

Fig. 2 **Central scotoma and visual distortion.**

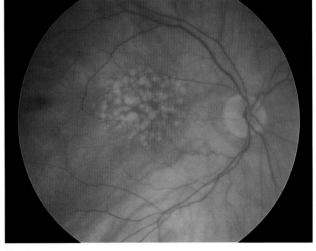

Fig. 3 **Drusen at the macula.**

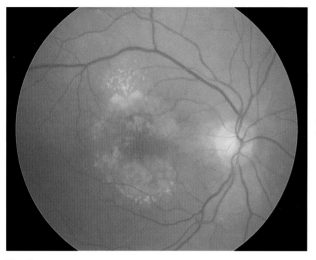

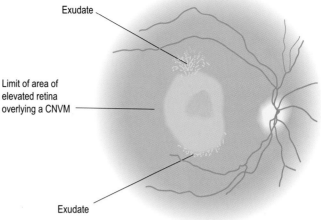

Exudate

Limit of area of
elevated retina
overlying a CNVM

Exudate

Fig. 4 **A choroidal neovascular membrane** (with explanatory drawing).

A CNVM may appear similar, but is often accompanied by haemorrhage and leakage of serum, with formation of exudate. Since this process usually occurs in a centrifugal fashion, the result is often a disc-like lesion with haemorrhage, drusen and RPE atrophy/hyperplasia at the centre and exudate and haemorrhage at the periphery (Fig. 4). Later, spontaneous involution occurs, leaving a large scar (Fig. 5) and severely impaired vision.

Prognosis
'Dry' AMD may progress very slowly, without significant visual loss but causing increasing difficulty with reading. In the 'wet' form, 75% of patients experience marked deterioration in vision over 3 years. Bilateral but asymmetrical disease leads to second eye involvement in 60% within 5 years.

Investigation
Fundus fluorescein angiography (FFA) is imperative when treatable choroidal neovascularisation is suspected.

Treatment
Although advances have been made in the last few years, active medical intervention remains of limited benefit.

Taking a high-dose antioxidant vitamin and mineral combination has been shown to have some effect, though limited, to modify the progression of macular degeneration in high risk patients. Counselling is important, particularly in patients with aggressive disease to whom it can be emphasised that navigable vision will be retained. Refraction, including the provision of low vision aids, is useful in maximising remaining visual function. Registration as blind or partially sighted may be appropriate.

A significant advance in treatment for 'wet' AMD has been the introduction of 'photodynamic therapy' (PDT), which involves the intravenous administration of a photosensitive agent selectively taken up by rapidly proliferating endothelial cells in the CNVM. Activation by a non-thermal 'cold' laser produces cytotoxic reactive oxygen species ('free radicals') that lead to thrombosis and involution of the CNVM (Fig 6). Treatment may have to be repeated every 3 months for about 2 years. Other forms of laser, irradiation and a range of surgical approaches have met with varying degrees of success and remain under investigation.

It is important to address coexistent pathology such as cataract and glaucoma.

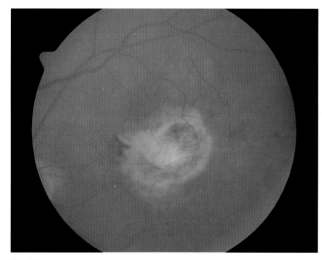

Fig. 5 **Macular scarring secondary to CNVM.**

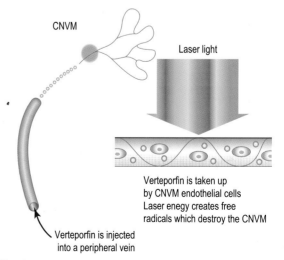

CNVM

Laser light

Verteporfin is taken up
by CNVM endothelial cells
Laser enegy creates free
radicals which destroy the CNVM

Verteporfin is injected
into a peripheral vein

Fig. 6 **Verteportin treatment of CNVM in maculas degeneration.**

Ocular fundus: macular disease II

Other disorders

Macular disorders typically disturb central vision but spare peripheral vision. This disturbance can be mild to severe.

Macular hole

Macular hole, an idiopathic loss of neural tissue at the centre of the macula occurring in the elderly, was previously thought to be a form of macular degeneration. Shrinkage and traction of the vitreous in front of the macula leads to the formation of a hole (Fig. 1). It is usually unilateral. Like AMD it causes loss of central vision only and does not lead to retinal detachment. Surgical removal of the vitreous (vitrectomy) and closure of the hole by gas tamponade, with or without application of autologous platelets, can result in improvement in sight.

Central serous retinopathy (CSR)

This occurs when the outer blood–retinal barrier (see p. 5) breaks down, permitting fluid to pass from the choroidal vasculature into the subretinal space. It is most common in young male adults and is unilateral. Visual acuity is mildly reduced, perhaps to 6/9. The retina at the fovea features a dome-shaped elevation which is difficult to identify other than by slit lamp examination (Fig. 2). Fluorescein angiography is diagnostic. Spontaneous recovery is usual, though often some reduction in visual function persists. The breakdown in the blood–retinal barrier can be closed by laser treatment, but at risk of damaging the delicate foveal photoreceptors.

Cystoid macular oedema (CMO)

Fluid *within* the retina, as opposed to *under* it (Figure 3), coalesces into cystic-looking spaces, disturbing the function of the neurosensory retina. Persistence results in irreversible sight reduction. It can be detected by careful binocular stereoscopic examination using the slit lamp and special magnifying fundus lenses, but fluorescein angiography is usually necessary to confirm its presence. The angiographic features (leakage of dye in a petal-like distribution) are typical and are different from those of age-related macular degeneration and central serous retinopathy.

The chief causes are diabetic maculopathy and retinal vein occlusion, but it is also the main reason for sight loss in uveitis, especially involving the posterior parts of the eye. It can also occur after cataract surgery, even when surgery is uncomplicated.

Treatment depends on the cause. Laser treatment of diabetic maculopathy can arrest disease progression but does not usually improve sight. The oedema of retinal vein occlusion may reduce after laser treatment, but often without paralleled gain in vision. When uveitis or cataract surgery is the cause, locally administered steroids, topically or by orbital injection, can restore sight. However, the longer the oedema is present, the more likely it is that sight reduction will be permanent.

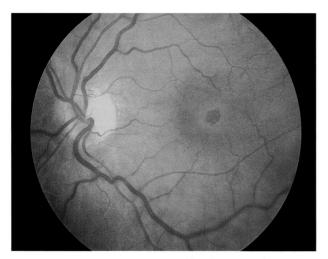

Fig. 1 **Macular hole.**

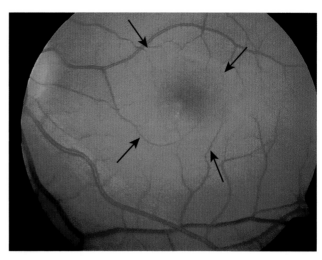

Fig. 2 **Central serous retinopathy. Arrows indicate the edge of the dome-shaped elevation.**

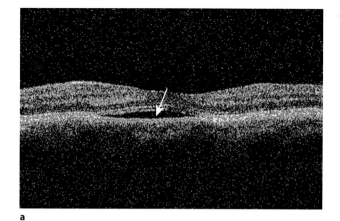

a

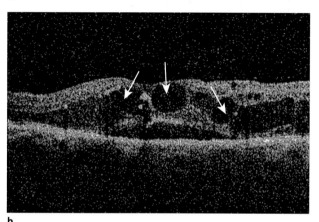

b

Fig. 3 **Optical coherence tomographs of CSR and CMO.** (**a**) subretinal fluid in CSR (arrow). (**b**) intraretinal cystic fluid spaces in CMO (arrows).

Epiretinal membranes (ERM)

The interface between the vitreous body and the retina can be the site for the development of a transparent contractile membrane. The typical feature is dragging of retinal vessels towards the fovea (Fig. 4); the result is reduction in visual acuity, sometimes with symptoms of distortion. Chief causes are diabetic retinopathy, retinal vein occlusion, uveitis, retinal detachment surgery and peripheral retinal tears. There may be no identifiable cause at all (idiopathic). The membrane can be peeled from the retina during vitrectomy surgery.

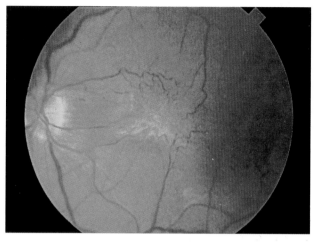

Fig. 4 **Epiretinal membrane, showing dragging of the perimacular blood vessels and fibrosis.**

Ocular fundus: macular disease

- Bilateral and age-related.
- Central scotoma on field testing.
- Normal pupil reactions.
- Changes localised to macula.
- Counselling is important.
- Refraction, low visual aids, register as visually impaired.
- 'Dry' AMD:
  – slowly progressive visual loss
  – drusen, mottled areas of pigment loss and increase
  – non-urgent referral.
- 'Wet' AMD:
  – distortion; sudden onset visual loss
  – haemorrhage and exudate
  – prompt referral.

Fluorescein angiography is usually necessary to confirm and characterise disease at the macula.

Macular hole
- Occurs in the elderly.
- Loss of neural tissue at the fovea.
- Causes distortion and/or loss of visual acuity.
- May be treatable with vitrectomy surgery.

Central serous retinopathy
- Occurs in young males.
- Fluid accumulation at the fovea.
- Mild reduction in visual acuity.
- Usually spontaneous resolution.

Cystoid macular oedema
- Fluid accumulation into cystic spaces within the neural retina.
- Chief causes are diabetic maculopathy, retinal vein occlusion, uveitis and cataract surgery.

Epiretinal membranes.
- Drag vessels towards the fovea.
- Can be peeled off.

Ocular fundus: hereditary disease

Retinitis pigmentosa

Retinitis pigmentosa (RP) describes the retinal appearance found in a variety of hereditary progressive degenerations of the retina. The ocular abnormalities may be an isolated finding or may be part of a systemic condition.

Degeneration of the rod photo-receptors is more marked than that of the cones.

Isolated primary retinitis pigmentosa can be sporadic or can be inherited in an autosomal recessive, autosomal dominant or X-linked pattern. There are many genetic subtypes of RP, resulting in a wide variation in age of onset and disease severity.

A number of non-hereditary conditions may mimic RP although they may affect only sectors of the retina:

- trauma
- retinal detachment surgery
- infections, e.g. syphilis, rubella
- previous occlusion of a retinal artery or vein
- drugs, e.g. chlorpromazine.

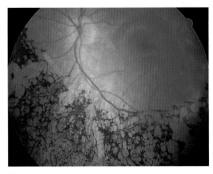

Fig. 1 **Bone-spicule pigmentation in RP.**

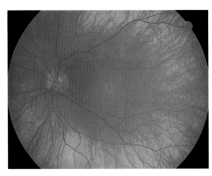

Fig. 2 **The albino fundus is hypopigmented.**

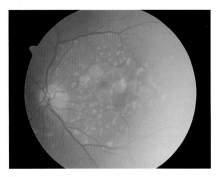

Fig. 3 **Retinal flecks in fundus flavimaculatus/Stargardt's disease.**

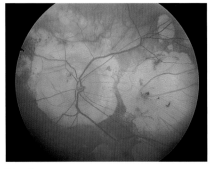

Fig. 4 **Chorioretinal atrophy in myopic degeneration.**

Clinical features
The chief symptoms are:

- night blindness ('nyctalopia')
- decreased peripheral vision
- decreased central vision (from macular changes)
- glare (from cataract).

'Bone-spicule' pigment clumping in the mid-periphery of the retina is characteristic (Fig. 1). Retinal arterioles become narrowed and the optic disc assumes a pale 'waxy' appearance. Cataract and cystoid macular oedema may develop, substantially reducing central vision.

Management
Electophysiological tests (ERG, EOG) assist in diagnosis. A detailed **family history** from as many blood relatives as possible is essential to help determine the mode of inheritance, which has important implications for predicting the course of the visual loss and for genetic counselling. Testing for the many genetic abnormalities associated with the clinical picture of RP may be carried out.

Associated systemic disease, which may be treatable, should be identified, particularly in children.

Prescription of low vision aids and support from social services can be very important. Cataract extraction may significantly improve visual function. Oral acetazolamide has been tried for the macular oedema of RP, with limited success.

Systemic associations of retinitis pigmentosa
There are a large number of systemic diseases and syndromes in which a pigmentary retinopathy is a component.

- **Usher's syndrome.** RP with congenital deafness (the most frequent cause of combined deafness and blindness in childhood).
- **Bassen–Kornzweig syndrome.** This disorder of lipid metabolism (also known as abetalipoproteinaemia) causes ataxia, red cell abnormalities and steatorrhoea. Treatment with vitamin A is beneficial, so early diagnosis is crucial.
- **Refsum's disease.** This is a polyneuropathy (including deafness) and cerebellar dysfunction resulting from abnormal phytanic acid metabolism. This disorder is also

treatable, by exclusion of phytanic acid from the diet. Presentation in adolescence or even adulthood with visual symptoms is usual.
- **Kearns–Sayre syndrome.** This is a triad of chronic progressive external ophthalmoplegia, cardiac conduction abnormality and pigmentary retinopathy, transmitted via abnormal mitochondrial DNA.
- **Leber's congenital amaurosis.** A form of early onset atypical RP, this may be associated with neurological and other systemic abnormalities.

Congenital stationary night blindness (CSNB)
CSNB is a generic term for night blindness, which, unlike RP, does not progress. The retina usually appears normal but electrophysiological tests show abnormal dark adaptation. A variety of CSNB, fundus albipunctatus, is characterised by multiple white spots in the peripheral fundus.

Cone dystrophy
In cone dystrophy there is progressive deterioration in the function of the cone retinal photoreceptors. Since cones are concentrated at the macula and provide colour vision, central

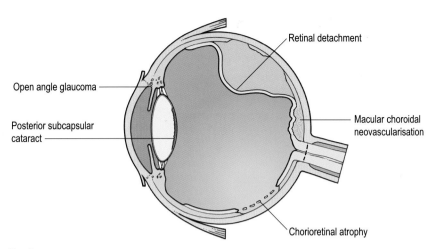

Fig. 5 **Ocular features associated with myopia.**

visual loss and loss of colour appreciation are the presenting complaints. Atrophic changes at the macula may be very subtle. Inheritance is usually autosomal dominant. Electrophysiological tests are essential in diagnosis.

Albinism

Failure of normal synthesis of melanin characterises albinism, which may be ocular or oculocutaneous. Inheritance may be autosomal recessive or X-linked.

Ocular features include congenital nystagmus, decreased visual acuity, strabismus, hypopigmented iris and pallor of the fundus (Fig. 2). Macular hypoplasia is invariably present.

The optic chiasm is anomalous, the majority of fibres from each eye crossing into the opposite optic tract.

Pale skin and hair are usually evident. However, genetic mosaicism in X-linked disease causes a spectrum of phenotypes, and affected individuals may go undiagnosed for many years. Mosaicism also accounts for asymptomatic retinal changes in carriers.

Stargardt's disease and fundus flavimaculatus

Also known as flecked retina, because of the appearance of creamy-white flecks (Fig. 3), these untreatable conditions cause loss of central vision during adolescence. The macula may be atrophic. Inheritance is usually autosomal recessive.

Electrophysiological assessment may be normal, especially in early disease. There is a characteristic appearance on fluorescein angiography: the 'dark choroid' effect.

Best's dystrophy

There is gradual accumulation in childhood of a yellow material at the macula which resembles the yoke of an egg (hence the alternative term vitelliform dystrophy). The EOG is always abnormal. There is no specific treatment. Inheritance is autosomal dominant.

Vitreoretinal dystrophies

Inherited retinoschisis

Retinoschisis (splitting of the retina) may be inherited (congenital) or acquired. The inherited type is an X-linked recessive condition. It causes a cystic appearance to the fovea of both eyes, from which radial striae extend over the macula in a bicycle-spoke pattern. In some patients the nerve fibre layer separates from the external retina in a sector of the peripheral fundus and becomes elevated within the vitreous cavity. Detached retinal vessels may bleed into the vitreous. Electrophysiological tests are abnormal.

Retinoschisis sometimes leads to true retinal detachment.

Stickler's syndrome

Stickler's syndrome is an autosomal dominant disorder in which skeletal abnormalities are associated with high myopia and vitreoretinal degenerative changes that predispose to retinal detachment.

Choroidal dystrophies

Myopia

High myopia, which has a strong familial tendency, is frequently associated with the development of progressive widespread chorioretinal atrophy (myopic degeneration) (Fig. 4). There may be night blindness and peripheral visual field loss. Often there is progressive macular atrophy and even choroidal neovascularisation, with severe central visual loss (Fig. 5).

Choroideremia

This X-linked recessive dystrophic disorder of the choroid causes progressive night blindness in childhood, followed by peripheral visual field loss and eventually central visual loss. There is progressive patchy peripheral chorioretinal atrophy. No specific treatment is available.

Gyrate atrophy

Gyrate atrophy is an autosomal recessive inborn error of ornithine metabolism. As with choroideremia, presentation is in childhood with night blindness and progressive visual field constriction. Scalloped patches of chorioretinal atrophy start in the periphery.

Dietary manipulation and pyridoxine (vitamin B6) supplementation is beneficial.

Ocular fundus: hereditary disease

- Key diagnostic points: nature of symptoms, family history, retinal appearance, associated systemic features, electrophysiological tests, fundus fluorescein angiography.

- Management: specific measures rarely possible but counselling, low visual aids and social support are all vital.

- Associated treatable ocular pathology such as cataract can occur.

- Retinitis pigmentosa is the most common inherited retinal condition. Ophthalmoscopic features include bone-spicule retinal pigmentation, waxy disc pallor, attenuated vessels and cystoid macular oedema.

- Retinopathy caused by a treatable systemic disease (e.g. abetalipoproteinaemia and Refsum's disease) should not be missed.

- High myopia predisposes to retinal detachment, chorioretinal atrophy, cataract, glaucoma and macular choroidal neovascularisation.

Ocular fundus: retinal detachment

The retina comprises two layers:

- the neurosensory retina, including the photoreceptors and the ganglion cell layer
- the retinal pigment epithelium.

A retinal detachment is a cleavage in the plane between the neurosensory retina and the retinal pigment epithelium (the subretinal space). Most cases of retinal detachment are rhegmatogenous, caused by a tear or hole in the neurosensory retina, which allows fluid from the vitreous humour to pass through into the subretinal space (Fig. 1). Degenerative changes in the vitreous are important in the pathogenesis of rhegmatogenous retinal detachment.

Retinal detachment without a retinal break (nonrhegmatogenous) may also occur (Fig. 1):

- tractional, when the retina is pulled off by membranes growing across its surface (e.g. advanced diabetic eye disease)
- exudative, caused by breakdown of the blood-retinal barrier allowing fluid to accumulate in the subretinal space (e.g. choroidal tumour, uveitis).

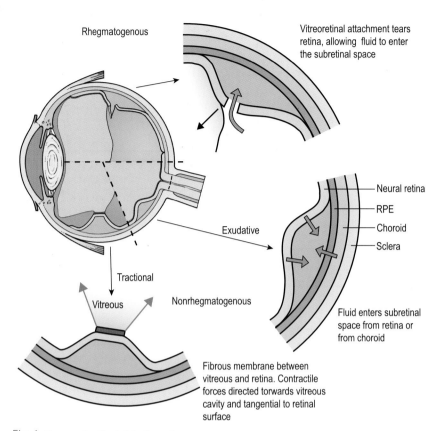

Fig. 1 **Causes of retinal detachment.**

Vitreous detachment

The vitreous humour is a gel consisting of water and glycosaminoglycans. It is structured, having a central body and a peripheral cortex. The cortex coats the retinal surface and in places is firmly attached to the retina. As part of the normal ageing process of the eye, the vitreous loses its gel structure and peels away from the retina (posterior vitreous detachment). Traction on the retina may then create a tear. This is more common in high myopes and following ocular trauma (blunt or perforating).

Symptoms

Posterior vitreous detachment (PVD) is very common. It causes floaters and flashing lights. The floaters are vitreous opacities and, sometimes, haemorrhage from torn retinal vessels. The flashing lights are caused by traction on the retina. Usually the floaters and flashing lights are a nuisance only, and reduce with time.

Management

No specific treatment is available, but the patient with an acute onset of vitreous detachment (less than 6 weeks) should be referred for dilated retinal examination, particularly if myopic.

Rhegmatogenous retinal detachment

Clinical features

- floaters/flashing lights
- peripheral field loss
- loss of central vision
- loss of red reflex
- detached retina.

Usually there is an antecedent history of vitreous detachment, but the importance of the symptoms may go unrecognised, so that presentation with visual loss is usual.

Early detachment of the retina causes loss of peripheral vision with preservation of normal central visual acuity. However, this may go unnoticed until the detachment reaches the macula. If the fovea detaches, central vision deteriorates badly, to 'hand movements'.

The peripheral field loss can be detected by simple confrontational testing. On fundal examination, detached retina is grey and the normal red reflex is lost. The grey retina seems to balloon forwards, requiring examination with 'plus' lenses in the ophthalmoscope. Retinal blood vessels are seen on the surface (Fig. 2). The degree of loss of vision and of red reflex depends on the area of retina detached.

Management

The only treatment is surgery (Fig. 3). Patients should be referred to an ophthalmologist immediately. The principles are:

- relief of vitreoretinal traction
- closure of the retinal break
- drainage of subretinal fluid
- adhesion of detached retina to retinal pigment epithelium.

Relief of traction can be achieved by removal of vitreous (vitrectomy) or by indenting the eye wall from the outside (placement of a sutured explant). This helps to close the break, which can be augmented by injection of gas or silicone oil. Drainage of subretinal fluid is achieved via a needle puncture through the sclera and choroid. External cryotherapy or internal laser causes inflammation of the choroid and retina and leads to adhesion of the neurosensory retina to the retinal pigment epithelium.

Prognosis

Visual recovery depends on the duration of retinal detachment and whether or not foveal detachment occurred. If the detachment is a few days old only, the prognosis is good. Surgery is usually successful, but reoperation is sometimes necessary, particularly if scar-like membranes

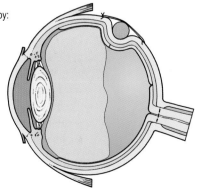

Fig. 2 **Retinal detachment.**

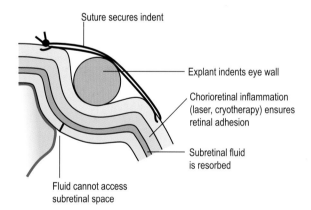

Suture secures indent
Explant indents eye wall
Chorioretinal inflammation (laser, cryotherapy) ensures retinal adhesion
Subretinal fluid is resorbed
Fluid cannot access subretinal space

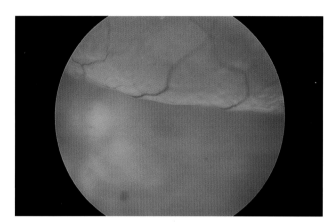

Vitreoretinal traction reversed by:
• indentation of eye wall (shown here)
• removal of vitreous (vitrectomy)

Fig. 3 **Retinal surgery.**

grow across the retina, pulling it off (proliferative vitreoretinopathy or PVR).

Tractional retinal detachment

Contractile membranes may grow across the retina in association with rhegmatogenous retinal detachment (see above) and in proliferative diabetic retinopathy. This kind of retinal detachment is especially difficult to treat. Optimal management of diabetic retinopathy should prevent this severe complication.

Serous (exudative) retinal detachment

The blood–retinal barrier comprises the junctions between adjacent retinal pigment epithelial cells (outer barrier) and the tight junctions of the endothelial cells of the retinal vasculature (inner barrier). Breakdown of the barrier may lead to intraretinal oedema and subretinal fluid (Fig. 1). Chief causes are:

n posterior uveitis
■ intraocular tumours
■ central serous retinopathy, affecting the macula.

Clinical features

These will include the features of any underlying disease and will depend upon the part of the retina involved. Usually only macular involvement will be symptomatic. The retinal detachment is much less extensive than with rhegmatogenous detachment (both in area and in volume) and may not be detectable on direct ophthalmoscopy.

Management and prognosis

Management depends on the cause. Spontaneous reattachment may occur. Foveal detachment will usually result in a degree of permanent impairment of visual acuity.

Acquired retinoschisis

This very common peripheral retinal degeneration is present in up to 1 in 10 of the population, more commonly in hypermetropes. As in inherited retinoschisis, an inner retinal layer becomes elevated. Though usually stable, it can occasionally progress to retinal detachment, for which it is sometimes anyway mistaken.

Ocular fundus: retinal detachment

■ Main cause is a break in the retina, associated with posterior vitreous detachment: requires surgical reattachment.

■ Floaters and flashing lights are caused by vitreous degeneration and vitreoretinal traction.

■ The red reflex is lost, the degree dependent on the area of detachment.

■ Peripheral visual loss initially will progress to loss of central vision when the detachment reaches the macula.

■ Retinal detachment without a retinal break is much less common; main causes include proliferative diabetic retinopathy, uveitis, intraocular tumours.

Optic disc swelling and optic atrophy

Many different processes may damage the optic nerve and impair vision, including disease of the central nervous system. Thus, patient assessment will often result in referral to a neurologist, occasionally as a matter of urgency.

These disease processes collectively usually result in vision loss, but clinical examination of the optic nerve head may show any of the following:

- no abnormality
- optic disc swelling: a non-specific term which includes papilloedema (Table 1)
- optic atrophy: a term used to describe an optic nerve which has lost substance, seen as a pale disc
- optic disc cupping: a characteristic of a specific disease entity (glaucoma).

Aetiology

It is convenient to consider causes anatomically (Fig. 1):

- within the globe
- within the nerve and sheath
- outside the nerve but in the orbit
- intracranial nerve (pre-chiasmal, chiasmal and post-chiasmal).

Pathogenesis

True papilloedema is a swollen optic nerve head due to raised intracranial pressure (Fig. 2). It is the result of impairment of normal axoplasmic flow. Disc swelling without raised intracranial pressure may be due to impairment of axoplasmic flow (as occurs in ischaemic and compressive states), oedema or infiltrate (Fig. 3).

Clinical features

These can be considered as:

- features of optic nerve dysfunction
- features of underlying disease
- associated findings.

Optic nerve dysfunction

The primary function of the optic nerve is vision, including visual acuity, peripheral vision and colour vision.

Visual acuity should be tested and recorded. Most disease processes cause loss of acuity, usually at an early stage. However, papilloedema causes late loss of acuity. Earlier, transient visual obscuration (blurring) is common.

Many types of field defect may occur. The swollen optic disc may cause enlargement of the blind spot only but the characteristic field defect is the

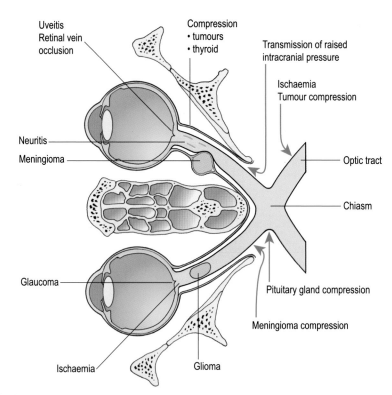

Fig. 1 **Causes of optic nerve disease.**

Table 1 **True disc swelling versus pseudopapilloedema**		
	Swelling	Pseudopapilloedema
Disc margin	Blurred	Clearly defined
Vessels	Blurred/obscured Congested veins	Clearly defined, no congestion
Cup	Early preservation	Frequently absent
Haemorrhages	Flame haemorrhages at disc margin are common	Absent
Cotton wool spots	Common	Absent

central. Other field defects, such as altitudinal loss, arcuate scotomas and hemianopias, usually occur due to specific pathologies causing damage at certain lacations along the course of the visual pathways. Thus, the altitudinal defect is typical of ischaemia at the optic nerve head, the arcuate scotoma occurs in glaucoma, the bitemporal hemianopia is caused by chiasmal disease and a homonymous hemianopia may be due to optic tract disease.

Confrontation testing using fingers or a red hat pin will usually be sufficient to detect a field defect. Formal perimetry can be used and may be useful in monitoring disease progression and treatment.

Red-green defects are typical of optic nerve dysfunction, so a bright red target, looking for desaturation (greyness), or Ishihara plates, should be used.

The swinging flashlight test may reveal a relative afferent pupil defect (pp. 15, 75).

Underlying disease

History and examination should consider raised intracranial pressure, ischaemia, systemic hypertension and thyroid disease. Ischaemia is associated with atherosclerosis, diabetes mellitus and giant cell arteritis. Many drugs are associated with benign intracranial hypertension and some, such as ethambutol, may cause optic atrophy. Optic atrophy is also associated with alcoholism. Intraocular inflammation may lead to optic disc swelling and late atrophy.

Associated findings

Raised intracranial pressure may cause a sixth nerve palsy (convergent squint with abduction weakness). This is a nonlocalising sign, meaning that the disease is not directly affecting the nerve, but indirectly causing it to be stretched or compressed. Proptosis indicates orbital disease. Flame-shaped

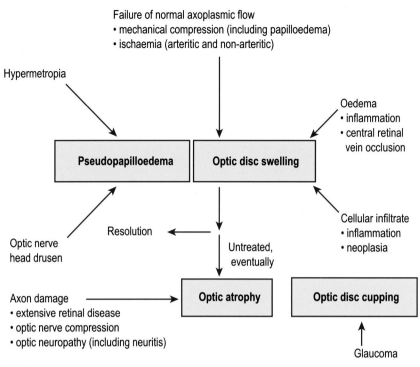

Failure of normal axoplasmic flow
- mechanical compression (including papilloedema)
- ischaemia (arteritic and non-arteritic)

Hypermetropia

Oedema
- inflammation
- central retinal vein occlusion

Pseudopapilloedema

Optic disc swelling

Resolution

Optic nerve head drusen

Cellular infiltrate
- inflammation
- neoplasia

Untreated, eventually

Axon damage
- extensive retinal disease
- optic nerve compression
- optic neuropathy (including neuritis)

Optic atrophy

Optic disc cupping

Glaucoma

Fig. 2 **Pathogenesis of optic nerve swelling and atrophy.**

retinal haemorrhages are characteristic of retinal vein occlusion.

Optic neuritis

The chief cause is demyelination; less common causes include viral infection and vasculitis.

The diagnosis is clinical. Chief features are rapidly progressive loss of vision (acuity and colour) in one eye with pain exacerbated by eye movement.

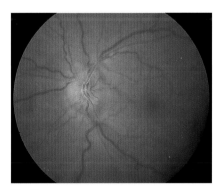

Fig. 3 **Acute papilloedema.**

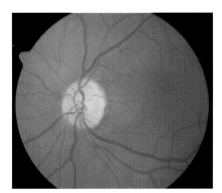

Fig. 4 **Optic atrophy.**

Field testing shows a central scotoma and there is a relative afferent pupil defect. The optic disc is usually normal, but may become swollen; following resolution, optic atrophy becomes apparent. Atypical features, such as fellow eye involvement, failure to recover and severe pain, warrant investigation.

Vision spontaneously improves almost to normal after a few weeks, even without treatment. The risk of development of multiple sclerosis is 60% at 5 years.

Anterior ischaemic optic neuropathy (AION)

Sudden onset sight loss, usually unilateral at first, may be preceded by transient episodes of vision loss. There is a relative afferent pupil defect and a swollen optic disc, with haemorrhage and cotton wool spots. Field loss is usually altitudinal. Two types are recognised: arteritic and nonarteritic. The arteritic form is caused by giant cell (temporal) arteritis. Urgent diagnosis and treatment with systemic steroids is necessary to prevent bilateral blindness. Key features are scalp tenderness with inflammatory swelling of the temporal arteries, jaw claudication and an elevated ESR and C-reactive protein level. (The latter *must* be measured *before* administration of systemic steroid). Biopsy of the temporal artery can be helpful. Systemic steroid use may need to be continued for several years to prevent relapse.

Nonarteritic ischaemic optic neuropathy has no sign of inflammation and is associated with atherosclerosis, hypertension, smoking and diabetes mellitus.

Pseudopapilloedema

'Pseudopapilloedema' is a nonpathologically swollen optic nerve. Hypermetropia (long-sightedness) is the most common cause. Optic nerve head drusen (hyaline bodies) is included, perhaps mistakenly since it may cause progressive field loss.

Investigations

Choice of initial investigation will depend on clinical findings, but will usually include neuroimaging (CT or MRI scan) at an early stage. Fluorescein angiography can help to distinguish true disc swelling from pseudopapilloedema, and an ultrasound scan will demonstrate optic nerve head drusen. Visual-evoked responses are used in the assessment of patients with demyelination.

Optic disc swelling and optic atrophy

Assess visual function including acuity, fields, colour vision, pupils.

Optic disc swelling
- papilloedema in raised intracranial pressure
- raised intracranial pressure causes transient blurring only
- papilloedema requires early neuroimaging
- other causes of disc swelling reduce the visual acuity
- other causes include direct compression, ischaemia, retinal vein occlusion, inflammation and infiltration
- beware pseudopapilloedema.

Optic atrophy
- loss of nerve fibres
- reduction in all parameters of visual function
- may indicate chronic intracranial pathology, nerve or intraocular disease
- consider neuroimaging.

Intraocular tumours

Retinoblastoma

Retinoblastoma is much the most common primary malignant intraocular tumour to affect children, with a frequency of 1 in 20 000. Presentation is usually at the age of about 18 months. Approximately 6% of patients have a family history of the tumour, which is transmitted via a gene on chromosome 13 as an autosomal dominant trait with 80% penetrance. In sporadic cases, 25% involve a new germline mutation which is, therefore, transmissible to offspring. Screening of siblings and offspring is vital.

The development of a white pupil (leukocoria, Fig. 1) in a small child is highly suggestive of retinoblastoma; the differential diagnosis is given in Table 1. The tumour usually appears as a whitish fleshy mass, which may be extremely large at presentation. Alternatively, it may grow beneath and elevate the retina. Strabismus and secondary glaucoma may occur.

Investigation

This should confirm the diagnosis and establish the presence and extent of extraocular spread, which may occur by local invasion and by haematogenous and lymphatic dissemination. Ultrasound, CT and MRI of the globe and orbit demonstrate the tumour and may show characteristic calcification. Serology may exclude a toxocara granuloma. Blood tests for a variety of tumour markers are sometimes positive. Systemic assessment for metastasis includes imaging, lumbar puncture and bone marrow aspiration.

Management

Large tumours are treated by removal of the eye (enucleation). Radiotherapy and chemotherapy are useful in some circumstances, often as an adjunct to enucleation.

Prognosis

The extent of optic nerve invasion will determine prognosis. A tumour confined to the globe is associated with a survival rate of over 90% at 3 years. Invasion beyond the neural transection point, however, carries a poor prognosis.

A second primary malignancy, such as a peripheral sarcoma, will develop in 10% or so of patients.

Choroidal naevus and melanoma

A variety of pigmented lesions can occur in the fundus (Table 2).

A **choroidal naevus** is a grey-brown flat or slightly raised discrete oval area. Most are less than three disc diameters across. They are very common and may be found in as many as one in ten of the general population. There is a small danger of malignant change, so suspicious lesions should be examined periodically, but population-based serial examination of all naevi is not practical and is unnecessary.

The choroid is the site of about 80% of uveal **melanomas**, the remainder developing in the iris or ciliary body. Choroidal melanoma (Fig. 2) is the most common primary intraocular malignancy to affect adults. The average age at presentation is 50 years.

Clinical features suggestive of malignancy include visual symptoms such as flashing lights (photopsia), substantial elevation, adjacent exudative retinal detachment, the presence of orange pigment deposits and increasing size.

Investigation

Systemic physical examination and investigation is performed to detect distant spread. Ocular ultrasound is the most useful imaging technique, aiding in diagnosis, assessment of tumour size and in the detection of trans-scleral extension.

Management

This is controversial and individual. Eyes with very large tumours usually require enucleation. In certain patients, treatments to preserve the globe are used: proton beam radiotherapy, radioactive plaque application and local resection. Where distant spread has occurred, palliative chemotherapy is considered.

Prognosis

This is extremely variable, dependent primarily upon tumour size (particularly thickness), histological

Table 1 **Causes of leukocoria**
Cataract
Toxocara granuloma
Retinoblastoma
Advanced retinopathy of prematurity
Vitreous maldevelopment (persistent hyperplastic primary vitreous)
Retinal dysplasias
Corneal opacity

Table 2 **Pigmented fundus lesions**
Choroidal naevus
Malignant melanoma
Hyperplasia of the retinal pigment epithelium
Secondary to chorioretinal degeneration, inflammation, infection
Deep haemorrhage (from a choroidal neovascular membrane)
Choroidal metastases
Age-related macular degeneration

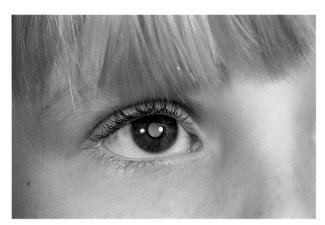

Fig. 1 **Leukocoria.**

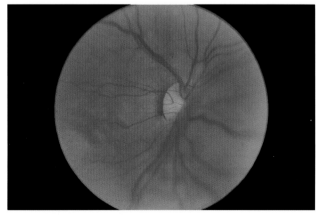

Fig. 2 **Choroidal melanoma.**

cell type and the presence or absence of detectable systemic metastasis.

Ciliary body and iris melanoma

Fifteen percent of uveal melanomas occur in the ciliary body. They may present with secondary glaucoma or uveitis or with manifestations of their local mass effect. The prognosis is worse than that of most choroidal melanomas, partly because they are detected at a later stage than more posterior lesions. Smaller ciliary body tumours can be removed by local surgical resection.

Approximately 5% of uveal melanomas affect the iris. In contrast to ciliary body melanomas they tend to behave in an indolent fashion; distinction between iris naevi and malignant lesions often depends on documented increase in size. Sector iridectomy usually achieves a cure.

Choroidal metastasis

Most malignant choroidal tumours are metastases from distant sites. It is likely that many go undetected in patients with disseminated cancer. Common sites of origin in adults are the breast, lung and gastrointestinal tract.

Metastases appear as pale shallowly elevated masses, often at the posterior pole and often multiple and bilateral. They frequently grow rapidly. Management options include: treatment of the primary tumour, observation (especially if asymptomatic) and palliative radiotherapy or chemotherapy.

Choroidal haemangioma

Discrete choroidal haemangiomas are seen as shallow dome-shaped orange-red lesions with overlying patchy retinal pigment epithelial changes. An exudative retinal detachment may be present adjacent to the lesion, and may be the cause of symptoms leading to presentation.

Asymptomatic haemangiomas are observed. Gentle laser is applied to the tumour if exudate threatens vision.

A morphologically distinct diffuse form of choroidal haemangioma occurs in association with Sturge–Weber syndrome (see below).

Choroidal osteoma

This is a rare benign yellow-orange calcified tumour near the optic disc of young women that may threaten vision by associated choroidal neovascularisation.

The phacomatoses

The phacomatoses (neuroectodermal syndromes) are a group of conditions characterised by neuroectodermal hamartomas involving multiple organs. Ocular manifestations are common.

Neurofibromatosis

Neurofibromatosis (NF), or von Recklinghausen's disease, is the most common phacomatosis. It is now known that there are at least two genetically distinct forms of the disease, NF 1 (peripheral) and the rare NF 2 (central, associated with bilateral acoustic neuroma and cataract). Both are transmitted in an autosomal dominant pattern.

Ophthalmic findings in NF 1 include proptosis, usually secondary to an orbital tumour (neurofibroma, meningioma or optic nerve glioma). Congenital or later onset glaucoma may occur. Multiple melanocytic hamartomas on the iris surface (Lisch nodules) are pathognomonic of NF 1.

Central and peripheral nervous system neurofibromas are common. Cutaneous lesions are the most obvious clinical manifestation; among the more frequent are fibroma molluscum (nodular overgrowths of neural connective tissue, often extremely numerous), axillary freckling and

pigmented patches known as cafe-au-lait spots. Bone dysplasia, scoliosis, cardiomyopathy and phaeochromocytoma may also occur.

Von Hippel–Lindau syndrome

In von Hippel disease haemangiomas arise on retinal capillaries, usually in the mid-peripheral fundus. These initially appear as tiny red dots which gradually enlarge to become nodular (Fig. 3). Vision is affected by leakage of blood or exudate. Lesions should be ablated by laser or freezing. In von Hippel–Lindau syndrome, cerebellar and visceral lesions are also present. Inheritance is sporadic or autosomal dominant. Family members should be screened.

Sturge-Weber syndrome

A cutaneous facial haemangioma ('port-wine stain') in the trigeminal nerve distribution is the most obvious sign of this nonhereditary condition, but patients also have a similar meningeal lesion. This may cause focal epilepsy and mental retardation. There may be a haemangioma of the outer sclera (associated with a secondary glaucoma) and diffuse choroidal lesion on the same side as the skin changes.

Tuberose sclerosis

Ocular lesions are found in about 50% of patients with this autosomal dominant/sporadic condition. The common finding is the retinal astrocytoma, a white lesion morphologically resembling a mulberry, usually at the optic disc. Systemic features include central nervous system astrocytic hamartomas, a variety of cutaneous abnormalities (adenoma sebaceum, shagreen patches, amelanotic patches, café-au-lait spots) and visceral hamartomas such as renal cysts. Epilepsy and/or mental retardation occur in a majority of patients.

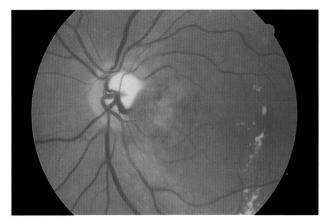

Fig. 3 **Retinal capillary haemangioma.**

Intraocular tumours

- Retinoblastoma is the most common primary intraocular malignancy in children; curative treatment is often possible; screening of siblings and offspring is essential.

- Intraocular melanoma is the most common primary intraocular malignancy in adults; choroidal form occurs most frequently; it is treated by enucleation or a range of conservative measures.

- Choroidal metastases indicate widespread dissemination from, commonly, breast, lung, GI tract; treatment is palliative, usually for symptomatic lesions only.

- Phacomatoses are a group of syndromes featuring multiple neuroectodermal hamartomas with many systemic features.

Strabismus: childhood

Strabismus, or squint, is a misalignment of the two eyes. If strabismus develops during the 'sensitive' period of visual development (up to 7–8 years of age), the brain responds by refusing to see (suppressing) the image from the deviating eye. This prevents double vision but leads to a condition known as amblyopia ('lazy eye'). Onset of strabismus after the sensitive period will usually result in double vision. The deviating eye may drift in any direction though certain patterns, particularly horizontal, are more common.

Terminology

Strabismus may be constant or intermittent and may vary with the direction of gaze.

- **Latent and manifest deviations.** A *latent* deviation is one which is controlled by subconscious effort: in certain situations, such as fatigue, control is lost and the deviation becomes *manifest*. A latent squint is a *-phoria*, a manifest deviation a *-tropia*.
- **Position of the eyes looking straight ahead.** When the eyes are convergent, the deviation is *eso-*; when the eyes are divergent, the deviation is *exo-*. Less commonly there is a vertical deviation (*hypo-* or *hyper-*). Eso-, exo-, hypo- or hyperdeviations may be manifest (-tropia) or latent (-phoria). Torsion (twisting of the eye) occurs rarely.
- **Angle of squint in different directions of gaze.** If the angle of the squint is the same in all directions of gaze, it is said to be *concomitant*; if not it is *incomitant*.
- **Eye movements.** Horizontal movement towards the nose is **AD**uction; **AB**duction is a lateral movement. Vertical movements are *elevation* and *depression*.

Childhood squints are usually concomitant, and eso- deviations predominate over exo-.

Amblyopia

During the sensitive period of visual development, permanent neural connections between the eye and the visual cortex are established. Amblyopia occurs when these connections are not completed. However, it is possible to encourage normal development with appropriate treatment during the sensitive period.

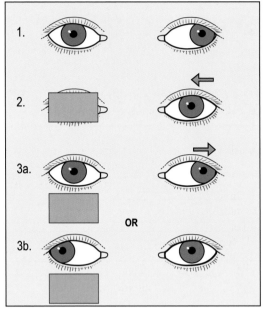

1. Right eye fixes on target

2. Left eye moves nasally to fix on target

3a. Right eye is uncovered, left eye moves laterally to original position

OR

3b. In alternating strabismus, the left eye maintains fixation, right eye is now divergent

Fig. 1 **The cover test (divergent strabismus).**

Amblyopia is characterised by reduced visual acuity (despite full correction of any refractive error) in the absence of any other organic explanation for reduced vision. The diagnosis is one of exclusion: an explanation for visual loss should always be sought.

Amblyopia is most commonly due to squint. Refractive error, particularly if asymmetrical (anisometropia), is another common cause and amblyopia will follow even reversible visual deprivation (e.g. cataract) during the sensitive period. Amblyopia is usually unilateral.

Although the cosmetic appearance of strabismus may be most distressing to child and parent, amblyopia is the more significant long-term consequence.

Binocular vision

Binocular vision is more than simply seeing equally well with each eye: at its highest level it enables stereopsis, an advanced form of three-dimensional sight.

Abnormal head posture

Incomitant deviations are often compensated by the involuntary adoption of a compensatory abnormal head posture. In this position, the angle of deviation is least and binocular vision may be achieved.

Assessment

The history should be directed at determining the age of onset and causative factors such as maternal infection, birth trauma, illness and family history. Neurological disease, including raised intracranial pressure, should be considered.

Measurement of visual function is more difficult the younger the child. A variety of simple and sophisticated techniques have been developed. The presence of strabismus is confirmed by the cover test (Fig. 1). The angle of deviation is measured using the cover test and prisms. Examination of the eyes in different positions of gaze helps to demonstrate abnormalities of ocular movement. Refraction, usually under cycloplegia (paralysis of accommodation), is essential. Binocular function can be tested. All children presenting with a squint should undergo a retinal examination with the pupils dilated.

Treatment

Treatment follows the scheme:

1. **Correct any refractive error.** This is usually with glasses. Normal visual development depends on seeing a clearly focused image. Spectacles are the usual means of correction and are generally worn continuously during waking hours.
2. **Reverse the amblyopia.** Occlusion of the better seeing eye forces the amblyopic eye to take up fixation and see. If amblyopia is severe, occlusion may not be tolerated: non-compliance

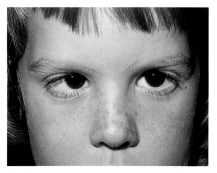 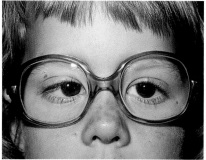

Fig. 2 **Convergent squint corrected with hypermetropic spectacles.**

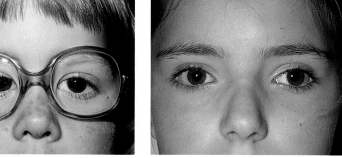

Fig. 3 **Left divergent squint.**

is a significant problem. Occlusion is usually part-time.

3. **Orthoptic management.**
Orthoptists have a major role in the assessment, diagnosis and monitoring of strabismus and visual development. Orthoptic treatment may help control intermittent and latent deviations.

4. **Surgery.** Altering the pull of the extraocular muscles by surgery cannot improve vision or reverse amblyopia, although parents may expect otherwise. Satisfactory cosmesis is often the only objective. Relief of an abnormal head posture is the next most common reason. More than one operation may be necessary, whatever the indication.

Most operations are weakening procedures (recession) which turn the eye away from the muscle, or strengthening procedures (resection) which pull the eye towards the muscle.

Convergent strabismus

Apparent (pseudo-) convergence is common, especially in the very young, and is usually due to a wide nasal bridge and vertical folds of skin at the medial canthus (epicanthic folds).

Two chief groups of true convergence are seen: infants with 'congenital' esotropia and children with later onset convergence. In infants the deviation may alternate between the two eyes. As a result, amblyopia is less likely but normal binocular development is impaired. Significant refractive error is uncommon. Surgery is performed in the second year. Children of 3 to 5 years may begin to overconverge as they increasingly focus on near objects (accommodative esotropia). This is typically associated with hypermetropia. Wearing glasses may fully correct the squint and restore normal vision (Fig. 2). Amblyopia requires occlusion therapy; any remaining squint can be corrected by surgery.

Rare causes of childhood convergent squint include Duane's syndrome and sixth nerve palsy. Duane's syndrome is failure of abduction (occasionally adduction) associated with retraction of the globe on adduction. Children often present with an abnormal head posture. Amblyopia is rare, and surgery can usually be avoided. A sixth nerve palsy may occur congenitally or may be acquired, sometimes due to raised intracranial pressure.

Divergent strabismus

This may be primary, secondary to organic visual loss or consecutive to a convergent deviation.

Primary exotropia begins intermittently, during fatigue, day-dreaming or staring into the far distance (Fig. 3). It may be associated with myopia. Binocular vision may be maintained by controlling the deviation, but if it is threatened, surgery may be required.

Divergence secondary to visual loss is more common than convergence, because of a 'natural' latent divergence.

Consecutive exotropia is a divergent squint which occurs after convergent squint surgery, usually many years later.

Other childhood oculomotor problems

Strabismus, nystagmus and other abnormalities of ocular movement are common in the presence of central neurological disease such as cerebral palsy and hydrocephalus.

A superior oblique weakness due to birth trauma may pass unrecognised for many years, until an abnormal

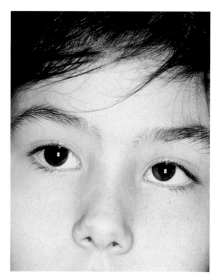

Fig. 4 **Abnormal head posture due to a superior oblique weakness.** The left eye is elevated (note the corneal light reflexes); the face is tilted to the right.

head posture and symptoms of eye strain and double vision occur (Fig. 4).

Brown's syndrome is a rare abnormality of superior oblique movement: the tendon fails to run smoothly through the trochlea, so that the eye cannot elevate in adduction.

Overaction of the inferior oblique muscle, causing the eye to shoot upwards in adduction, is commonly present with estropia. A weakening operation can be combined with surgery for the convergent deviation.

Many of the 'adult' causes of strabismus, such as myasthenia gravis, orbital fracture, myopathy and nerve palsy, may also occur in children.

Strabismus: childhood

- Main causes: idiopathic, refractive error, visual loss, central or peripheral neurological deficit.
- Main consequences: amblyopia, lack of normal binocular vision, poor cosmesis.
- Convergent squint: early-onset, non-refractive; later onset, usually with hypermetropia; Duane's syndrome.
- Divergent squint: idiopathic; myopia; secondary to visual loss.
- Treatment: correct refractive error; reverse amblyopia (occlusion therapy); surgery.

Strabismus: adult

Strabismus or 'squint' is an ocular misalignment. It should not be confused with the layman's understanding of 'squint', meaning to 'look through screwed up eyes'.

Although there is overlap between childhood and adult strabismus, a practical differentiation is made for two reasons: (1) onset after the sensitive period (up to about 7 years of age) usually causes double vision; (2) adult strabismus is usually caused by disease of the efferent limb of the control of ocular alignment.

Aetiology

Ocular alignment depends on an intact afferent input (sight), an intact efferent pathway (nerves and extraocular muscles) and normal processing and control centres in the brain. All causes of strabismus can be considered in this afferent–central–efferent organisation, and the history, examination and investigation should be directed accordingly:

- afferent
  - visual loss
- central
  - decompensation of childhood squint
  - disturbance of processing and control centres
- efferent
  - cranial nerves 3, 4 and 6
  - neuromuscular junction
  - extraocular muscles.

Patient assessment

History

The chief symptom is double vision: two images seen clearly but separately from each other. This should be differentiated from blurred vision and from monocular multiple images (usually caused by cataract). If double vision is caused by ocular misalignment, it will resolve if either eye is closed. The double vision may be intermittent, especially if disease severity varies or if ocular alignment changes with direction of gaze. Double vision can be horizontal, vertical or diagonal, depending on the position of the two eyes relative to each other, and will suggest the aetiology.

Squint without double vision implies suppression by the brain of the image from one eye. This usually occurs in childhood squint but can also be 'learned', as a means of overcoming double vision.

The history should include questions about general medical problems and symptoms of neurological disease.

Examination

First, check the visual acuity then verify ocular misalignment.

Ocular position

Strabismus is confirmed by the cover test (Fig. 1) using the corneal light reflex.

Ocular movement

Precise examination of ocular movement requires considerable practice and experience, but a simple examination should be attempted. Use a target such as a pen torch, which allows you to see asymmetry of the corneal light reflex. Move the target slowly and methodically in an 'H' pattern, asking about double vision. Lack of movement and maximal double vision in a particular position will suggest the muscle/nerve that is at fault.

Complex patterns are usually caused by widespread extraocular muscle weakness, e.g. myasthenia gravis and dysthyroid eye disease.

Ocular examination

This is particularly important if vision is poor. Look for opacities (especially

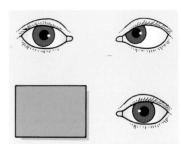

1. The right eye is fixing; the left eye is convergent.

2. When the fixing right eye is covered, the left eye makes an outward movement to take up fixation (movement may not be detected if deviation is small or, if vision is poor, eye may not move to fixate).

3. Query if double vision resolves when one eye is covered.

Fig. 1 **The cover test** (convergent strabismus).

cataract), and at the fundus (optic disc swelling or atrophy, retinal disease).

Orbital examination

Look for signs such as ptosis, lid retraction and lid lag on downgaze. Proptosis (protruding eye or eyes) suggests a mass in the orbit. 'Mass' can include the swollen extraocular muscles of dysthyroid eye disease.

Further examination.

The history and examination should have resulted in a differential diagnosis after which tests for specific diseases and further examination can proceed.

Specific diseases

Visual loss

Unilateral visual loss, usually due to cataract or retinal disease, causes the brain to lose afferent feedback in its attempt to control the position of the two eyes.

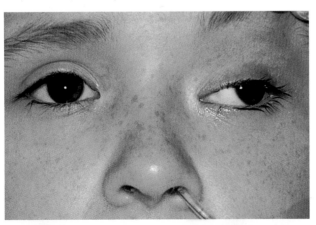

Fig. 2 **Left third nerve palsy** (the ptotic lid is being lifted).

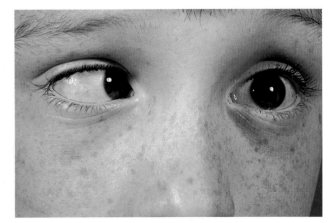

Fig. 3 **Left sixth nerve palsy** (eyes gazing to the left).

Decompensation of childhood squint

The childhood squint, which may or may not have been operated on, might always have been obvious (manifest strabismus) or may have been controlled (latent strabismus) by fusional forces which later fail. The failure, and consequently the double vision, may be intermittent.

Nerve palsies

The third, fourth and sixth cranial nerves run a long course, from brainstem to orbit, and may be damaged at any point (Table 1).

Third nerve damage will usually cause divergence, ptosis and pupil dilation (Fig. 2), though an ischaemic cause will often lack pupillary involvement. Recovery may occur but can be incomplete or aberrant.

It is difficult to examine for the consequences of fourth nerve damage. Diplopia will be vertical or diagonal, and may be torsional. Usually, no cause is found: mild head trauma is the most common reason. The prognosis for recovery is good.

Palsy of the sixth nerve is easy to diagnose. The eye is convergent and fails to turn laterally (abduction weakness) (Fig. 3). Again the prognosis is good.

Neuromuscular junction

Myasthenia gravis is an autoimmune disease in which antibody blocks the acetylcholine (muscarinic) receptor at the neuromuscular junction (Fig. 4). The autonomic system is not involved. The effects may be entirely ocular, but very often other muscle groups are involved. Typically symptoms are variable, worse with effort and worse at the end of the day. The autoantibody can be detected in serum. Electromyography is also helpful. Treatment is outlined in Figure 4; immunosuppression with steroids and azathioprine may be required.

Extraocular muscles

Dysthyroid eye disease is usually associated with hyperthyroidism (Graves' ophthalmopathy), but any thyroid state may be present. Infiltration of the extraocular muscles and of the soft tissue within the orbit by inflammatory cells with associated oedema causes proptosis and muscle weakness. The muscle problems vary with time and are rarely stable, so that corrective surgery is unpredictable. Prisms fitted to spectacles can be helpful.

Nonspecific orbital inflammation may cause a myositis.

Inherited orbital myopathy (chronic progressive external ophthalmoplegia, or CPEO) is a disorder of mitochondrial DNA, which is inherited from the

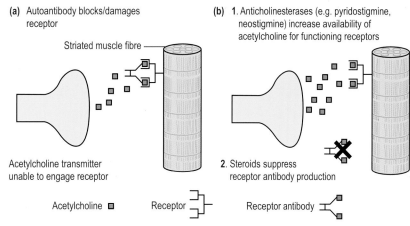

Fig. 4 **Cause (a) and treatment (b) of myasthenia gravis.**

mother. Muscle involvement is symmetrical, so that diplopia is unusual. Bilateral ptosis also occurs. Ptosis props fitted to spectacles and ptosis surgery may be helpful, but extraocular muscle surgery should be avoided. Other features include a retinal pigmentation that resembles retinitis pigmentosa, epilepsy and heart block.

A blow-out fracture of the orbital floor may cause entrapment of orbital tissue around the inferior rectus muscle. The eye on the affected side may be drawn downwards and fail to move up or down fully. Double vision is more likely to occur with up and down movement than in straight ahead gaze. Adequate recovery is frequent, but surgery may be needed if diplopia on downgaze persists.

Supranuclear disturbance of eye movement

Coordination of eye movement depends on pathways originating in the cerebral hemispheres, the cerebellum and the vestibular nuclei which travel to the horizontal gaze centre in the pons and to the vertical gaze centre in the midbrain. These are the 'supranuclear' controls of eye movement. The gaze centres project to the third, fourth and sixth cranial nerve nuclei.

A wide variety of eye movement disorders may occur as a result of disease of supranuclear controls. The most common pathologies are ischaemia, haemorrhage, tumours and demyelination.

Vertical gaze problems occur in lesions of the dorsal midbrain (Parinaud's syndrome) and in a Parkinson-like syndrome of progressive supranuclear palsy (Steele–Richardson syndrome).

Disruption of the medial longitudinal bundle, which connects centres for horizontal movement, results in an **internuclear ophthalmoplegia**. There is reduced adduction on the side of the lesion and nystagmus of the abducting fellow eye. It is especially associated with demyelination.

Table 1 **Causes of nerve palsies**
Idiopathic – usually spontaneous full recovery
Microvascular disease (hypertension, diabetes mellitus, atherosclerosis) – usually spontaneous full recovery
Trauma – even minor head trauma can cause a fourth nerve palsy
Aneurysm of the posterior communicating artery, causing a third nerve palsy with pain and pupil involvement
Inflammation – including any cause of vasculitis, sarcoid meningitis, Guillain–Barré syndrome and infections (herpes zoster, syphilis, TB)
Neoplasia – benign or malignant, primary or secondary, by compression, usually without evidence of raised intracranial pressure

Strabismus: adult

- Strabismus, or squint, means misalignment of the eyes.

- In adults, diplopia (double vision) is usually the main symptom.

- Confirm with cover test; examine ocular movements.

- Consider causes using afferent–central–efferent system:
  – afferent: visual loss
  – central: decompensating childhood strabismus
  – efferent: cranial nerves 3, 4 and 6; neuromuscular junction; extraocular muscle.

- Diseases of supranuclear controls most commonly caused by demyelination, ischaemia, haemorrhage.

- Internuclear ophthalmoplegia: ipsilateral adduction failure, nystagmus of abducting fellow eye.

Unequal and abnormal pupils

Pupillary abnormalities are not common but worry the clinician, who is concerned to avoid missing serious neurological disease.

The normal pupil

The normal pupil is located slightly nasal to the centre of the cornea. Fine oscillations in size and a small amount of asymmetry between the eyes (anisocoria) are usual. Physiological asymmetry persists whatever the ambient illumination. Pathological anisocoria varies between dark and light conditions.

Pupil size is determined by a balance between the sphincter muscle and the dilator muscle. The parasympathetic nervous system, carried in the third cranial nerve, innervates the sphincter muscle (Fig. 1). The synapse between pre- and postganglionic fibres is in the ciliary ganglion in the orbit, and the transmitter at the neuromuscular junction is acetylcholine. The sympathetic nervous system innervates the dilator muscle. The postganglionic fibres originate in the superior cervical ganglion in the neck and run a long course, including an intracranial component, to reach the orbit. The transmitter is noradrenaline.

Pharmacological tests of pupil function (Fig. 2)

Cocaine

Cocaine 4% prevents reuptake of noradrenaline from the neuromuscular junction into the sympathetic nerve ending (Fig. 2a). It will dilate the normal pupil but not a pupil in which there is loss of sympathetic innervation.

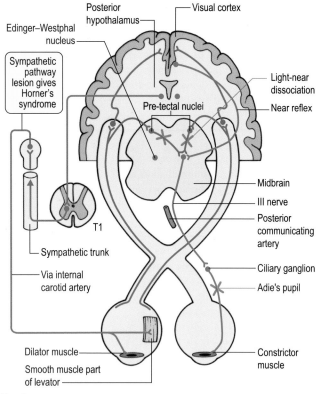

Fig. 1 **Pupil innervation, including some sites of pathology.**

Denervation hypersensitivity

When postganglionic fibres are damaged, there is a reduction of transmitter secretion and release. In response, the understimulated end-organ, in this case the iris muscle, develops an excess of receptor and becomes hypersensitive, such that it will react to only a small quantity of transmitter. This is known as denervation hypersensitivity (Fig. 2b).

Postganglionic parasympathetic lesions.

The pupil will constrict to 0.1% pilocarpine (a cholinergic agonist), whereas the normal pupil will be unaffected.

Postganglionic sympathetic lesions.

The pupil will dilate to 0.1% adrenaline, whereas the normal pupil will not.

Unequal pupils

Posterior synechiae

Intraocular inflammation (iritis) can lead to the formation of adhesions between the iris and the lens, known as posterior synechiae. The adhesions are only rarely complete, so the pupil margin becomes irregular in shape

(p. 46). This is most obvious when the pupil has been dilated. Light reactions should be normal but will be difficult to detect.

Acute glaucoma

During an attack of acute glaucoma, the intraocular pressure may become so high that ischaemic damage results, particularly at the 3 and 9 o'clock positions, causing the pupil to become vertically oval. It reacts poorly to light.

Third nerve palsy

A third nerve palsy causes a dilated pupil that fails to react to light or accommodation. The anisocoria is most obvious in bright light, when the normal pupil constricts but the abnormal pupil remains dilated. There should be other features of a third nerve palsy, such as ptosis and a divergent squint.

Third nerve palsies are differentiated into 'medical' and 'surgical': pupillo-motor fibres in the third nerve have a different blood supply from the rest of the nerve, so that in microvascular disorders such as diabetes mellitus pupil involvement is typically spared ('medical thirds'). 'Surgical' causes, such as an aneurysm of the posterior

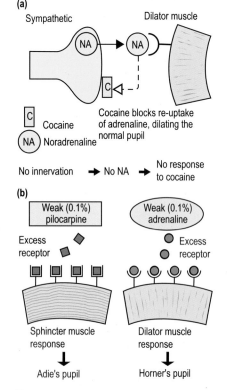

Fig. 2 **Tests of pupil function. (a) Loss of sympathetic innervation; (b) denervation hypersensitivity.**

communicating artery, characteristically involve the pupil.

Acute rise in intracranial pressure, after head injury for example, may cause a rapidly evolving third nerve palsy, manifested as a sudden dilation of the pupil. This has given rise to the phrase 'the pupils have blown'.

During recovery from a third nerve palsy, nerve fibre regeneration may be aberrant. Typically, there is pupil constriction on adduction of the affected eye.

Adie's pupil

Damage to the postganglionic parasympathetic fibres in the orbit causes a semidilated pupil that reacts poorly to direct light and to accommodation. Redilation is slow. The sphincter muscle can contract a little, particularly with prolonged stimulation. Under the magnification of the slit lamp, sectoral iris atrophy and worm-like contractions are seen. The disruption of accommodations may cause blurring of vision. With time, the affected pupil becomes miosed.

The cause is not known, but a viral aetiology is assumed. In some patients the deep tendon reflexes (such as at the ankle) are lost.

There is denervation hypersensitivity, so the diagnosis is confirmed by pilocarpine 0.1%.

Horner's syndrome

Horner's syndrome (Fig. 3) causes a miosis through damage to the sympathetic innervation, at any point along the pathway between the hypothalamus and the eye (Fig. 1). The anisocoria is most obvious in dim illumination, when the affected pupil fails to dilate naturally. Because the Müller's muscle component of the upper lid levator muscle is innervated by the sympathetic system, there will also be a mild ptosis. If the lesion occurs below the superior cervical ganglion, ipsilateral facial perspiration will be diminished and facial flushing will be present, although these features are usually transient. The light and near reflexes are not affected.

Congenital or infantile Horner's syndrome is associated with iris heterochromia.

Cocaine 4% dilates the normal pupil but not the Horner's pupil (Fig. 2a), whereas adrenaline 0.1% dilates only the Horner's pupil (denervation hypersensitivity, Fig. 2b).

Investigation is directed at the cause, especially since the sympathetic chain may be involved by lung cancer (Pancoast's tumour).

Other abnormal pupils

Light-near dissociation

This term describes pupils that react poorly or not at all to light but which constrict to a near stimulus. The causative lesion is in the midbrain, affecting the internuncial neurones which pass from the pretectal nucleus to the Edinger–Westphal component of the third nerve nucleus but sparing the near reflex pathway that bypasses the internuncial neurones (Fig. 1).

Argyll Robertson pupils, in neurosyphilis, are the best known example but are in fact rarely encountered. Both pupils are involved. They are usually small and irregular and dilate poorly. Neurosyphilis may also cause fixed dilated pupils.

Trauma, tumours, vascular malformations, infarcts, haemorrhages and demyelination may all cause light-near dissociation. An associated failure of upgaze and convergence–retraction nystagmus together constitute **Parinaud's syndrome**.

Light-near dissociation also occurs as part of diabetic neuropathy, in dystrophia myotonica and in aberrant third nerve regeneration.

The relative afferent pupil defect

A relative afferent pupil defect is best detected by the swinging flashlight test. The direct and consensual light reflexes mean that a light swung from one eye to the other and back again should result in pupils that stay equally constricted. However, if the afferent pathway on one side is damaged, the stimulus to constriction on that side will be reduced. When the light is swung from the normal to the abnormal side, there is less stimulation so that the pupil on the abnormal side appears to dilate, but reconstricts when the light is swung back to the normal eye.

As the light is swung from eye to eye, there is alternate constriction and dilation of each pupil.

The test requires a bright light source, much brighter than the standard pen torch or most direct ophthalmoscopes. It should be performed with the subject looking at a distant target, to avoid the confounding effect of accommodation. This point is often overlooked.

The test is positive in unilateral disease of the optic nerve, retinal detachment, severe 'wet' macular degeneration and, occasionally, in amblyopia, but negative in the presence of corneal opacity, cataract and vitreous haemorrhage, so it is an important diagnostic point in assessing visual loss.

Drugs

Mydriatics and miotics, if administered to one eye only, cause unequal pupils. Administration may be inadvertent.

Systemically administered anticholinergics, including atropine and many neurotropic drugs, may dilate the pupils. Opiates cause miosis.

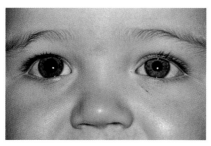

Fig. 3 **Left Horner's syndrome.**

> ### Unequal and abnormal pupils
>
> **Unequal pupils**
> - Posterior synechiae: irregular; normal reactions but difficult to detect
> - Acute glaucoma: oval, semidilated; poor direct light reflex
> - Third nerve palsy: dilated nonreactive pupil; associated ptosis and divergent strabismus; requires investigation
> - Adie's pupil: disorder of postganglionic parasympathetic fibres; slow irregular contraction; constricts to 0.1% pilocarpine
> - Horner's syndrome: disorder of sympathetic supply, pre- or postganglionic, at any point along the pathway; associated ptosis; requires investigation; no response to cocaine 4%; dilates to 0.1% adrenaline.
>
> **Light-near dissociation**
> - Disorder of internuncial neurones in the midbrain
> - Chief causes include neurosyphilis, infarction and haemorrhage, tumours and demyelination.
>
> **Drug**
> - Opiates cause miosis
> - Many neurotropic agents cause dilation.

Trauma: eyelids, orbits and head

The separation of eyelid and orbital trauma from that of the eyeball is convenient since it is common for the globe to be spared serious damage even when trauma to periocular structures is severe. Head trauma may cause direct ocular and orbital trauma or may indirectly impair visual function by, for example, injury to nervous tissue.

EYELID TRAUMA

Blunt trauma

Even minor blunt trauma can cause massive bruising ('black eye'), since the eyelid skin is so easily distensible. Applying ice may reduce the degree of swelling. It is not uncommon for blood to track across the nose and spread around the uninvolved eye, which may cause understandable concern.

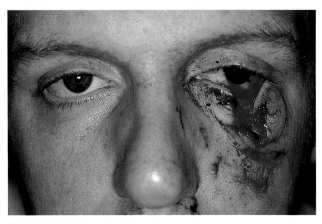

Fig. 1 **Lid margin laceration.**

Lacerations

Superficial lacerations of the skin and orbicularis oculi muscle which do not involve the lid margin heal well. During skin repair it is important to conserve tissue, even if it appears devitalised. The blood supply to the facial skin is so good that it is rare for it to undergo avascular necrosis.

Disruption of the lid margin (Fig. 1) and involvement of the levator muscle or medial canthus may cause permanent cosmetic and functional changes.

If the lid margin is cut, it should be repaired taking care to appose adjacent layers, especially in the upper lid (levator muscle) and at the medial canthus (medial canthal ligament). The grey line, which separates the line of meibomian gland orifices from the eyelashes, is a good anatomical marker. Each of these structures should be repaired in turn before tackling the skin laceration, which should then come together easily (Fig. 2). Lid margin sutures should be left in place for 10–14 days.

Damage to the levator muscle may cause a ptosis. Primary repair should be undertaken in layers, the identification of which may be difficult. Even after careful repair, ptosis may persist. Further surgery should be delayed for at least six months.

The lower eyelid is held against the globe by the medial canthal ligament, which links the tarsal plate with the lacrimal crest, located in front of the lacrimal fossa. Correct medial canthus positioning helps the collection of tears by the eyelid puncta but repair of this important ligament is often overlooked.

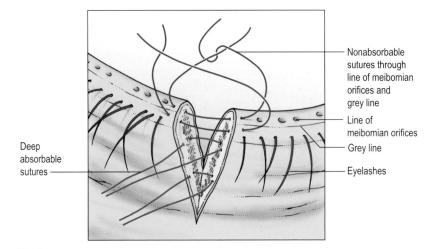

Deep absorbable sutures

Nonabsorbable sutures through line of meibomian orifices and grey line

Line of meibomian orifices

Grey line

Eyelashes

Fig. 2 **Lid margin repair.**

Canalicular laceration should be suspected when there is disruption of the medial canthus, particularly if the lid margin is involved. Canalicular repair requires special surgical expertise and is often unsuccessful. Fortunately, the presence of one intact canaliculus is usually sufficient to prevent a watery eye.

Skin contracture (cicatrisation) after trauma may cause ectropion. This can be corrected by scar excision and Z-plasty, which alters the direction of pull of contracting tissue. Rarely, skin grafting may be necessary.

Burns

The main consequences of eyelid burns, whether thermal or chemical, are tissue loss and contracture, which cause disfigurement and corneal exposure. The exposed cornea should be kept moist with chloramphenicol ointment and covered with transparent cooking wrapper, which reduces evaporation. Skin and mucosal grafting may be necessary.

ORBITAL TRAUMA

The bony orbital rims protect the eyes in most cases of facial and head trauma but are themselves rarely significantly fractured. However orbital 'blow-out' fracture is common and the orbital walls and rims may be involved in extensive facial fractures.

Blow-out fracture of the orbit

The orbit has a thin floor and a thin medial wall. Sudden rise in intraorbital pressure, as may occur when the eyeball is struck and propelled backwards, is likely to be 'decompressed' by fracture of these thin structures (Fig. 3). Alternatively, strong forces applied to the orbital rim may be transmitted along the orbital floor, which, as the weaker structure, fractures.

Clinical features

Fracture of an orbital wall increases the effective volume of the orbit. This results in enophthalmos (sunken eye), which may be masked in the early stages by orbital haemorrhage. The connective tissue around the adjacent rectus muscle may be trapped in the fracture site. Thus a fracture of the floor causes limitation of ocular elevation and depression, and limited horizontal movement occurs when the medial wall is fractured. Double vision results. This is most disabling in straight ahead and downward gaze.

The infraorbital nerve courses along the floor of the orbit. Damage leads to altered sensation of the cheek.

Surgical emphysema may occur as air passes from the paranasal sinuses through the fracture into adjacent soft tissues.

Plain X-rays may show a sinus 'fluid level' or opacification, owing to haemorrhage, and sometimes prolapse of orbital tissue into the maxillary sinus ('teardrop sign'), but confirmation of an orbital fracture usually requires a CT scan (Fig. 4).

Management

Systemic antibiotics should be prescribed as the fracture is, in effect, compound. The timing of surgical intervention is controversial, enophthalmos being the main indication. The ocular motility disturbance often resolves spontaneously as haemorrhage clears. When surgery is undertaken, the objectives are to free trapped orbital tissue and to cover the bony defect, usually with bone from another site, such as the skull, or with a synthetic plate.

Facial fractures

Major facial trauma tends to cause fractures in specific patterns within the facial skeleton. These have been described by Le Fort. Repair is complex and usually requires a multidisciplinary approach guided by CT scanning and three-dimensional image reconstruction.

HEAD TRAUMA

Massive head injury may cause direct damage to eyeball, lid and orbital structures. In addition, involvement of intracranial nervous structures can impair visual function by interrupting the visual pathway or by interfering with the control of eye position and movement. Rapid deceleration and shaking can cause additional damage.

Chief ocular consequences of head trauma are:

- vitreous haemorrhage
- optic nerve compression, section or avulsion
- macular oedema
- visual field deficit
- cranial nerve palsy
- loss of function of higher visual centres (visual association areas and control centres for eye movement).

A common consequence of even minor closed head injury (such as falling off a bicycle) is a fourth cranial nerve palsy. It causes double vision, especially diagonal and even torsional, which is most severe on looking down (reading, going up and down steps).

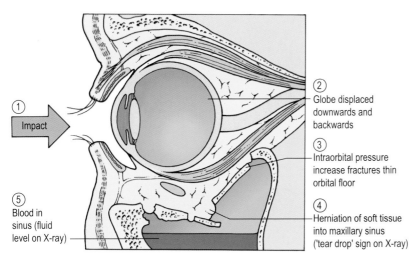

① Impact
② Globe displaced downwards and backwards
③ Intraorbital pressure increase fractures thin orbital floor
④ Herniation of soft tissue into maxillary sinus ('tear drop' sign on X-ray)
⑤ Blood in sinus (fluid level on X-ray)

Fig. 3 **Mechanism of blow-out fracture.**

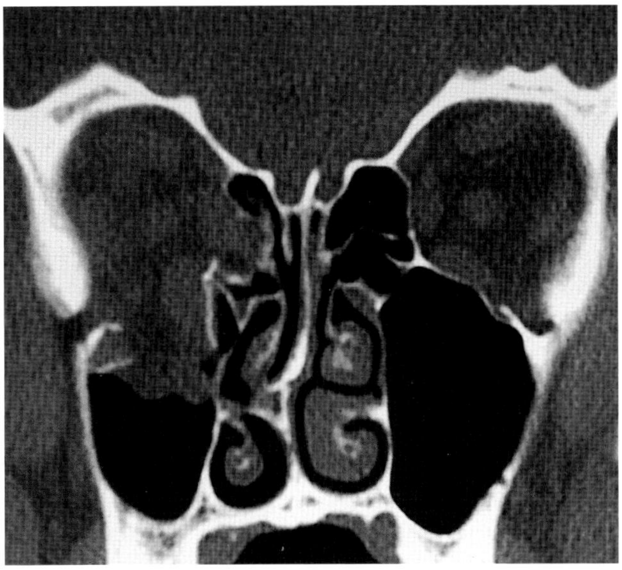

Fig. 4 **CT scan of right orbital floor fracture.**

Trauma: eyelids, orbits and head

Eyelid trauma
- Conserve tissue; repair in layers, especially the lid margin and levator muscle in the upper lid (to avoid ptosis).
- Consider the presence of eyeball or orbital trauma.
- At the medial canthus, canalicular laceration causes watering; medial canthal ligament avulsion requires repair.
- Risk of corneal exposure with tissue contracture or loss.

Orbital fracture
- Blunt trauma can cause orbital blow-out fracture.
- Signs include enophthalmos, infraorbital anaesthesia, reduced vertical eye movement.
- Diagnosis is confirmed with CT scan.
- Ocular motility disturbance frequently resolves. Treatment should include systemic antibiotics (compound fracture); enophthalmos may require surgical reconstruction.

Trauma: the eyeball

Trauma at home, in the workplace and during leisure pursuits is a significant cause of ocular morbidity and visual loss, particularly in the under-60s.

Patient assessment must include a careful history, especially if ocular perforation by high-velocity objects is not to be missed. *Visual acuity must be recorded.* Lid swelling may make ocular examination difficult, but it should be possible to part the lids with gauze, cotton-tipped buds or retractors. In the patient with multiple trauma, a brief examination of the eyes should not be forgotten. Equally, ocular examination must not detract from attention to cardiorespiratory status and the conscious level.

Physical trauma

Superficial trauma

Subconjunctival haemorrhage

Bright red blood looks dramatically serious as it spreads underneath the transparent conjunctiva but is usually insignificant, except when it masks a scleral perforation.

Corneal abrasion

This is demonstrated with fluorescein drops and a blue light: the dye pools in the defect and shines green (Fig. 1). Multiple pinpoint 'abrasions' may be caused by ultraviolet light (sunbeds, welding torches). Conventional treatment consists of chloramphenicol ointment with or without a cycloplegic (cyclopentolate 1% or homatropine 2%), for comfort, and occlusive padding for a day, followed by four times a day chloramphenicol ointment for 4–7 days.

Foreign bodies

These are usually cleared by the tear film but may lodge underneath the upper lid or embed in the cornea (Fig. 2). They cause intense irritation and profuse watering. Removal of subtarsal and superficial corneal foreign bodies is achieved using a cotton-tipped bud, after instillation of benoxinate or amethocaine anaesthetic drops. Embedded corneal foreign bodies are best removed with a hypodermic needle under magnification. If the bevel of the needle is directed parallel to the surface of the cornea, so that the edge of the bevel strikes the edge of the object, needle perforation of the cornea is impossible. Iron-containing foreign bodies may produce a rust-like ring around them, which is more difficult to remove. Once the foreign body has been removed, treatment is the same as for an abrasion, but intraocular penetration should be considered if a high-velocity impact has occurred. Secondary infection is very rare.

Blunt trauma

The orbital margins protect the eyeball from most blunt objects, but any large object striking the eye with force may cause considerable damage. **Hyphaema** (Fig. 3) is bleeding into the anterior chamber and always indicates that the eye has suffered sufficient trauma to cause significant damage to any intraocular structure. Vision may be reduced to seeing hand movements only but soon recovers as the blood clears. Ophthalmological examination, to detect trauma at other sites in the eye, is mandatory. It is usual to put the patient with hyphaema on bed rest, at home or in hospital, to avoid

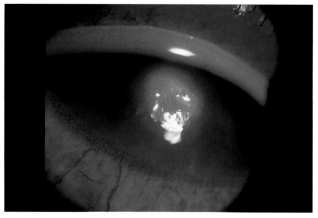

Fig. 1 **Corneal abrasion.**

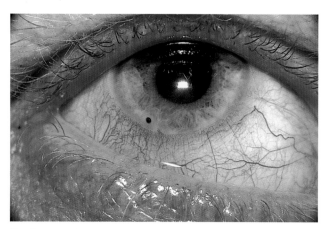

Fig. 2 **Corneal foreign body.**

a secondary haemorrhage. The blood comes from the anterior chamber angle or the iris, so **pupil abnormalities** (usually dilation or ovalling) are common and may be permanent. Retinal **commotio** (traumatic oedema) appears glistening white; it resolves without sequelae. Retinal tearing, leading to retinal detachment, and rupture of the choroid, usually at the macula, are fortunately rare, but are the main reasons for permanent visual impairment. **Rupture of the globe** is very rare. Vision is severely reduced and the red reflex is absent, owing to hyphaema and vitreous haemorrhage.

Perforating trauma

Intraocular foreign body

Although ocular perforation usually causes some degree of visual loss with hyphaema and even vitreous haemorrhage, a history of impact by a high-velocity foreign body without obvious sign of trauma should alert the examiner to the possibility of **intraocular foreign body**. The consequences of failure to identify a foreign body are major: intraocular infection in the short-term, retinal detachment in the medium-term and siderosis in the long-term. Therefore, X-ray or CT scan and ophthalmological referral are mandatory. Glass is inert, but copper causes an aggressive inflammation and iron-containing objects release ferrous ions into the eye (**siderosis**). Toxic ferrous ions are deposited in the retina (permanent visual loss), the iris (heterochromia), and trabecular meshwork (glaucoma).

Treatment of intraocular foreign bodies includes antibiotics and prompt removal, followed by expert care to maximise visual recovery. If the lens is damaged by the foreign body, cataract is inevitable.

Corneal and scleral lacerations

May be partial- or full-thickness. Uveal tissue, which is dark brown in colour, may prolapse through the wound (Fig. 4). Scleral wounds may be masked by haemorrhage. The objective in the repair of scleral lacerations is restoration of the integrity of the ocular wall. Careful repair of corneal lacerations is more important: scarring causes astigmatism and opacity, which will impair vision even when no other structure is involved. Scarring is more severe when repair is poorly completed.

Long-term consequences

Significant ocular trauma may have long-term consequences in addition to those immediately predictable from the nature of the injury.

The lens may be lost at the time of the injury, or may need to be removed because of **cataract** formation, which is common, even when the lens has not been directly damaged. Correction of aphakia with an intraocular lens may not be possible, necessitating contact lens use.

A secondary open angle **glaucoma** is common, caused by damage to anterior chamber angle structures. **Retinal**

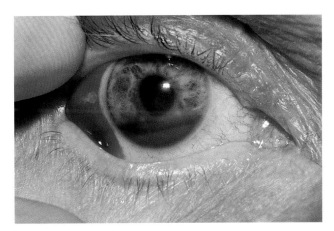

Fig. 3 **Hyphaema.**

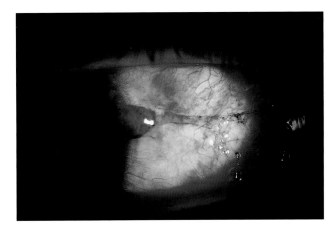

Fig. 4 **Corneoscleral laceration with iris prolapse.**

detachment caused by disinsertion of the retina at its anterior extremity, the ora serrata, may be only slowly progressive and may present years after the original injury.

Corneal scarring and astigmatism may require corneal transplantation. Corneal decompensation, through endothelial cell loss, may also result.

Loss of vision in one eye disrupts the central inputs required for control of ocular alignment, leading to acquired strabismus, usually divergent.

A severely injured eye may be chronically inflamed and uncomfortable, and may eventually require removal, even if not completely blind.

Perforation of the globe with exposure of uveal tissue may rarely be complicated by **sympathetic ophthalmitis**, an autoimmune reaction that attacks the healthy fellow eye. It can be prevented by early removal of the injured eye, which is especially indicated if it is completely blind (no light perception). Once sympathetic ophthalmitis has begun, historically the prognosis has been poor, but treatment with newer immunosuppressants has improved the outcome.

Chemical burns

The eyes can easily be involved in chemical trauma, by a variety of minor irritants (perfumes, hair sprays), and more harmful acids and alkalis (including detergents). Fortunately, most chemicals are irritant only, causing skin erythema and conjunctival injection, perhaps with punctate epithelial erosions. These pinpoint areas of fluorescein staining are usually located on the interpalpebral cornea and conjunctiva (unprotected by the eyelids).

Acids coagulate proteins so tend not to penetrate the eye. Alkalis, however, can cross cell membranes, penetrating the conjunctiva and the cornea and passing deep into the eye. Large areas of epithelial loss and limbal ischaemia (a measure of tissue damage), may result in corneal opacification and chronic ocular surface dysfunction. Glaucoma and cataract may also ensue.

Conjunctival scarring can lead to entropion and loss of tear-producing glands. Scarring of the skin may cause ectropion and corneal exposure. Such deformities exacerbate the ocular surface dysfunction.

Entropion and ectropion can be managed surgically, but with difficulty because of tissue loss and contracture.

Trauma: the eyeball

- A careful history is necessary to determine type of injury.
- Some assessment and record of visual acuity is mandatory.
- Subconjunctival haemorrhage is common and trivial, unless it masks perforation of the sclera.
- History of sharp trauma or high velocity impact should alert examiner to possibility of perforation; blinding siderosis is main consequence of undetected intraocular foreign body.
- Corneal abrasion heals rapidly without scarring; conventional treatment is chloramphenicol ointment and pad. Corneal foreign body is removed and then treated as for an abrasion.
- Hyphaema: rest from physical activity and await spontaneous clearance before examining the whole eye for other damage; associated pupil abnormality is common.
- Burns: alkali tend to be worse; irrigate fully, then assess degree of limbal ischaemia and corneal clarity as measures of tissue damage.

Neonatal conjunctivitis

Conjunctivitis which occurs during the first postnatal month is termed 'ophthalmia neonatorum'. Because the usual causes are specific to this age group, it is regarded as distinct from conjunctivitis occurring in older infants. In the United Kingdom, medical professionals are legally obliged to notify the local public health authority of all cases.

Investigation and management are modified according to the clinical picture. An ophthalmological opinion is generally indicated.

Aetiology

Microorganisms which may be acquired by the child during vaginal delivery include *Chlamydia trachomatis*, herpes simplex virus and *Neisseria gonorrhoeae*, associated with maternal sexually transmitted disease. However, staphylococci, streptococci and *Haemophilus influenzae* are also common causes of conjunctivitis in the neonate. Topical preparations, such as antiseptics, may cause conjunctival hyperaemia, mimicking infective conjunctivitis.

History

The interval between birth and the onset of inflammation provides a clue to the likely cause (Table 1). There may be a history of conjunctivitis in family members and other contacts. The parents should be questioned about symptoms of sexually transmitted disease. It is also essential to ask about systemic illness in the baby: chlamydia in particular may cause extraocular manifestations such as pneumonitis and otitis.

Examination

There may be variable degrees of eyelid redness and swelling (Fig. 1). Vesicles on the lid skin suggest herpes simplex. A purulent discharge is typical of gonococcal and other bacterial infections, whilst chlamydia usually causes a mucopurulent reaction. If no discharge is evident, a chemically-induced inflammation should be suspected. Adequate corneal inspection is difficult, due to floppy eyelids which tend to evert rather than open, but is mandatory: gonococcal keratitis, for instance, can progress rapidly to corneal perforation.

Severe inflammation can result in permanent conjunctival and corneal scarring.

Investigation

Conjunctival swabs are taken for microscopy, including chlamydial immunochemistry, and for chlamydial, bacterial and viral culture. A conjunctival scrape can be examined using special techniques for evidence of various infective agents. If chlamydia is suspected, swabs are also taken from extraocular sites such as the ears, throat and rectum.

Fluid from skin vesicles can be sent for viral culture.

It is important to refer the mother and her sexual contacts for investigation when a sexually transmitted infection is diagnosed.

Differential diagnosis

A watery eye with little redness and sticky discharge is often caused by congenital nasolacrimal duct obstruction rather than primary conjunctivitis.

It may be difficult to distinguish severe conjunctivitis from orbital cellulitis. Very occasionally, a bacterial conjunctivitis can develop into a cellulitis affecting the superficial tissues ('preseptal' cellulitis) or the orbit itself.

Treatment

If there is no corneal involvement and no rapidly progressive severe infection, a broad-spectrum topical antibiotic such as chloramphenicol or fusidic acid is appropriate.

Chlamydia is treated with oral erythromycin, for two weeks. (Oral tetracycline stains growing teeth and is therefore contraindicated in children.) Aciclovir, given via topical and systemic routes, is used in herpes simplex infection.

Bacterial conjunctivitis is managed with the appropriate antibiotic. The gonococcus is usually sensitive to benzylpenicillin or a cephalosporin.

If the diagnosis is uncertain and the infection severe and rapidly progressive, a range of samples is taken for investigation and treatment with a broad spectrum topical antibiotic such as cefuroxime (to ensure cover for gonococcus) is commenced. The baby is reviewed daily.

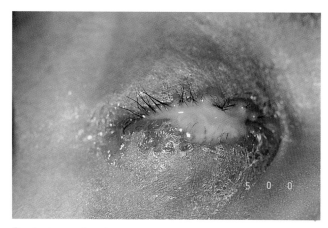

Fig. 1 **Neonatal conjunctivitis.**

Table 1 **Ophthalmia neonatorum: clinical features aiding differential diagnosis**

Aetiology	Presentation	Discharge	Maternal genitourinary Infection	Additional features
Chlamydia	1–3 weeks	Mucopurulent	Yes	Pneumonitis, rhinitis, otitis
Gonococcus	First week	Severe purulent	Yes	Keratitis if untreated
Herpes simplex	1–2 weeks	Watery	Yes	Lid vesicles, keratitis
Staphylococci and other bacteria	End of first week onwards	Purulent	No	Keratitis (rare)
Chemical	First few days	Nil/watery	Possible	

Neonatal conjunctivitis

- Conjunctivitis during the first postnatal month.

- Notifiable condition.

- Chief cause is chlamydia: oral erythromycin for 2 weeks.

- Chief mimic is congenital nasolacrimal duct obstruction.

- Frequently associated with maternal sexually transmitted disease.

- Be aware of possibility of extraocular disease.

Episcleritis and scleritis

Episcleritis and scleritis are inflammatory conditions involving the opaque ocular outer wall, the 'white' of the eye (see p. 3). They usually cause aching and redness which is more severe in scleritis than episcleritis (Table 1). The two conditions are almost certainly distinct entities.

Episcleritis

Episcleritis, a non-infective inflammation involving a thin tissue layer superficial to the sclera and deep to the conjunctiva, is extremely common, particularly in young adults. The hyperaemia can be segmental (Fig. 1) or, less often, diffuse and does not involve the palpebral conjunctiva. Pain is usually mild at most and may be absent. Unlike conjunctivitis, it does not cause discharge. Sight is not affected. Without treatment the condition is usually self-limiting, though weak topical steroid or non-steroidal anti-inflammatory drugs (NSAIDs) will settle any pain and speed resolution. Episcleritis is only rarely a manifestation of a systemic disease, in contrast to scleritis (see below).

Scleritis

Scleritis is generally a more serious condition than episcleritis, both in terms of the clinical features – severe

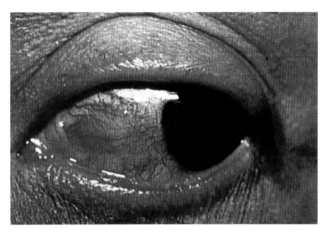

Fig. 1 **Episcleritis.** Segmental hyperaemia.

Table 1		
Feature	**Episcleritis**	**Scleritis**
Incidence	Common	Rare
Inflammation	Superficial; bright red	Deep; violet hue
Pain	Absent to mild	Moderate to severe
Associated systemic disease	Rare	Common
Visual disturbance	Extremely rare	Not uncommon

pain is often present – and the presence of associated systemic disease. The inflammation involves the full thickness of the sclera. Deeper, larger blood vessels can be seen to be engorged on slit lamp examination, and the inflammation more frequently involves the whole circumference of the anterior segment. Scleritis may be associated with scleral thinning; corneal thinning ('melting') and even perforation can also occur.

Scleritis involving the posterior part of the sclera may cause no redness of the front of the eye, but ultrasound scanning demonstrates the inflammation.

In at least half of patients with scleritis an underlying systemic inflammatory disease is present, including current or previous herpes zoster ophthalmicus, rheumatoid arthritis and systemic lupus erythematosus.

Treatment depends on severity, and may include topical and systemic steroids and NSAIDs. Severe cases may require immunosuppressive therapy.

Episcleritis and scleritis

Episcleritis
■ Red eye without pain, change in sight or discharge.

Scleritis
■ Very rare cause of a painful red eye.
■ Often associated with systemic disease.

Special topics in ophthalmology

Correcting refractive errors

Refractive errors occur when the optical system of the eye fails to focus an object onto the retina. The optical components of the eye are:

- the cornea
- the lens
- the length of the eyeball.

Of these, the cornea is the most powerful focusing element but only the lens is naturally adjustable. All three components change during childhood as the eye grows.

Normal refraction

In normal sight (emmetropia), light from a distant object is focused on the retina. As the object comes closer to the eye, the lens increases in power by altering its shape to become more convex (Fig. 1). This active process of accommodation is stimulated by parasympathetic fibres in the oculomotor nerve.

Refractive errors

An imbalance of the optical components of the eye leads to a refractive error (ametropia). In long-sightedness (hypermetropia or hyperopia), the refractive power of the eye is inadequate so that light from distant objects is focused 'behind' the eye. An additional convex lens is required (Fig. 2). In short-sightedness (myopia), distant targets are focused in front of the retina. This is corrected by a concave lens (Fig. 3). However, objects close to the myopic eye may be focused directly onto the retina: hence the term 'short-sightedness'.

In astigmatism, the power of the focusing elements is different in different meridians. For example, light from the top and bottom of an object may be focused in one plane, but light from its sides in another. In simplistic terms, the eye behaves like a rugby ball instead of a soccer ball. Correction requires a lens shaped like a rugby ball turned through 90 degrees (Fig. 4). Astigmatism may occur in addition to myopia and hypermetropia.

Refractive errors are common. In childhood, as the cornea and lens grow and the eye elongates, the initially hypermetropic eye may become emmetropic or even myopic. Myopia is especially common in oriental races.

Refractive errors may be iatrogenic. Cataract surgery is the most common cause for two chief reasons. Firstly, tension in sutures inserted to close the incision may distort the shape of the cornea, causing astigmatism. This can usually be reduced by suture removal, but some induced astigmatism may persist. This form of astigmatism is less common in modern 'small-incision' cataract surgery. Secondly, the refractive power of the removed human lens must be replaced.

Ageing changes

With increasing age (particularly after age 40 years), the deformability of the lens reduces, accommodation begins to fail and the point of closest focus falls further and further from the eye. This natural phenomenon is known as presbyopia. It is overcome by a convex lens (reading glasses, Fig. 5).

Increasing density of the lens nucleus (nuclear sclerosis) is a common variety of cataract. The increase in density is accompanied by an increase in refractive power, which can lead to the development of myopia in the elderly. Distant objects are less distinct and out of focus, but the ability to read unaided improves.

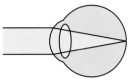
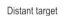
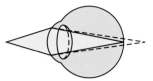

Distant target

Accommodation: increase in convexity of lens in order to focus near target

Fig. 1 **Emmetropia and accommodation.**

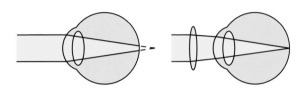

Hypermetropia (long sight): 'naturally' corrected by accommodation (increasing the refractive power of the lens) until presbyopia occurs

Fig. 2 **Hypermetropia.**

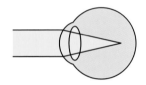

Myopia: concave lens required for distant focusing

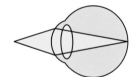

Light from near target is divergent, so is focused on retina, hence, 'short sight'

Fig. 3 **Myopia.**

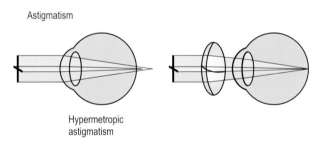

Astigmatism

Hypermetropic astigmatism

Fig. 4 **Astigmatism.**

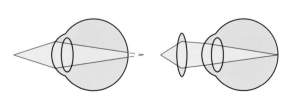

Presbyopia: convex lens assists focusing of near target

Fig. 5 **Presbyopia.**

Correcting refractive errors

Most refractive errors can be corrected by spectacles. The use of contact lenses is mostly for cosmetic reasons. The demand for refractive surgery, particularly to reduce myopia, is increasing.

Spectacles

Spectacles easily correct low degrees of ametropia. Modern manufacturing techniques produce lightweight highly effective inexpensive lenses. Inserted into a suitably selected frame, they become a projection of the individual's personality and even a fashion accessory.

Lenses for both near and distance vision can be inserted into a single frame (bifocals) or combined to produce a graduated lens for objects at any distance (varifocals). Anti-scratch and anti-reflective coatings with fixed and variable (photochromic) tints can be added.

Higher degrees of ametropia are more difficult to correct with spectacle lenses, or may be cosmetically unacceptable (Table 1).

Contact lenses

There are two major types: rigid and soft.

Rigid lenses come in two varieties: hard and gas permeable. These float on the eye separated from the cornea by the tear film, which conveys oxygen to the cornea for the maintenance of normal metabolism.

The gas permeable lens also allows oxygen to diffuse through the lens material to reach the tear film. In contrast, the soft lens lies directly on the corneal surface and so must be fully permeable to oxygen.

In general, soft contact lenses are more comfortable and are preferred by most users. Unfortunately, the incidence of serious complications is greater than with rigid lenses (Table 2). However, new silicone-based soft lens materials are likely to offer improvements to safety.

Meticulous lens care and hygiene are necessary to minimise problems (Table 3).

Surgery and laser

User dissatisfaction and inability to achieve best potential vision with spectacles and contact lenses has fuelled a rapid expansion in the availability and demand for surgical methods of refractive error correction.

Incisional techniques such as radial keratotomy alter corneal curvature but are now infrequently used for the correction of simple ametropia.

Incisional surgery does have a role in the correction of higher levels of astigmatism, for example, after corneal transplantation or during cataract surgery.

The excimer laser can be used to shave off ultra-thin layers of corneal tissue in order to reduce the refractive power of the cornea (photorefractive keratectomy or PRK) (Fig. 6). This technique has been incorporated into the 'LASIK' (LASer In situ Keratomileusis) procedure in which a flap of superficial cornea is cut and folded back and the exposed corneal surface is lasered. LASer-assisted subEpithelial Keratectomy (LASEK) is a modification of PRK in which the epithelium is pushed to one side as a single sheet. It is replaced after laser ablation. LASIK, LASEK and PRK have a high success rate so that patient satisfaction is high, but complications, though rare, can occur (Table 4).

Removal of the human lens in cataract surgery results in the state of aphakia. The most common method of correction is the intraocular lens implant, inserted at the same operation. An intraocular lens can be inserted as a secondary procedure. A range of intracorneal and intraocular implants have been introduced for the correction of refractive errors in the phakic eye, but are currently largely investigational.

Table 2 Complications of contact lens use

- Punctate corneal erosions secondary to epithelial ischaemia
- Corneal vascularisation
- Allergy to or toxicity from preservatives
- Giant papillary conjunctivitis (undersurface of upper lid – resembles hay fever)
- Corneal ulceration and infection

Table 1 Spectacles – limitations

Most spectacles are worn successfully. Problems occur with increasing refractive error.

- Cosmesis: convex magnify, concave minify
- Distortion of objects in peripheral vision
- Magnification of objects by highly convex lenses
- Weight
- Cannot correct severe astigmatism

Table 3 Contact lens care

- Do not exceed the recommended wearing time
- Observe meticulous hygiene
- Do not clean with tap water or saliva
- Remove if the eye becomes sore or inflamed
- Remove soft lenses while administering preservative-containing drops

---

Table 4 PRK, LASEK and LASIK

Benefits	Correction of myopia (–1 to –10 dioptres) and hypermetropia (+1 to +6 dioptres)
	High level of patient satisfaction
	Improvement in unaided visual acuity
Complications	Corneal haze
	Over-correction, under-correction
	Loss of best-corrected visual acuity
	Regression of effect
	Glare, haloes, starburst phenomena

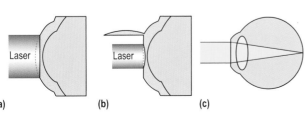

(a) (b) (c)

Fig. 6 **(a) Photoreactive keratotomy; (b) LASIK; (c) correction of myopia: flattening of the anterior corneal surface reduces its focusing power.**

Correcting refractive errors

- Hypermetropia (long sight) requires convex lens.
- Myopia (short sight) requires concave lens.
- Presbyopia (age-related failure of accommodation) requires convex lens.
- Spectacles correct most refractive errors.
- Contact lenses are useful for cosmesis and greater refractive errors but meticulous care is needed to avoid complications.
- Excimer laser surgery increasingly popular for refractive error correction.

HIV and the eye

Human immunodeficiency virus (HIV) infection is associated with a wide range of ocular disease. An ophthalmic presentation can sometimes be the first clinical evidence of immune dysfunction and may lead to the discovery of previously unsuspected HIV infection.

The course of HIV infection and AIDS is improving with the introduction of new therapies, such as combination regimes (e.g. HAART).

Ophthalmic diseases that occur in HIV infection often show a different pattern and follow a different course to that seen in immunocompetent individuals with the same conditions.

Disorders involving the eyes and adnexal structures are among the most common clinical manifestations of HIV infection. Often their presence indicates advanced disease. Severe visual loss is frequent as a result of:

- retinitis (cytomegalovirus, PORN toxoplasmosis)
- corneal disease (herpes simplex, varicella-zoster)
- uveitis (toxoplasmosis, syphilis)
- optic neuropathy (syphilis, lymphoma).

Eyelids

Kaposi's sarcoma appears on the skin as an unsightly dark red nodule or plaque that does not blanch with pressure (Fig. 1). Diagnosis is usually clinical but can be confirmed by biopsy. Local radiotherapy, chemotherapy and surgical excision are treatment options.

Several **infections** are seen with increased frequency and severity in HIV patients. Examples include chalazion, herpes simplex and ophthalmic shingles. Herpes simplex and zoster infections are both treated with systemic aciclovir.

Molluscum contagiosum, caused by a pox virus, is a whitish nodular lesion at the lid margin (Fig. 2). Viral material is shed into the tear film, causing a chronic conjunctivitis. In immunocompetent individuals the lesions are usually solitary and resolve spontaneously within a few months; the immunocompromised are prone to develop multiple persistent nodules.

Seborrhoeic dermatitis is common in HIV infection and this can be associated with blepharitis.

Conjunctiva

Conjunctival microvasculopathy, with capillary irregularity and flow abnormalities, is a universal finding in patients with AIDS. The precise mechanism is uncertain.

Dry eye is very common. Symptomatic patients are treated with simple ocular lubricants.

Kaposi's sarcoma of the conjunctiva is brighter red than that seen on the skin.

Cornea

Most forms of keratitis, including bacterial, fungal and viral, tend to be more common and more severe in the immunocompromised. The dry eyes and blepharitis frequently seen in HIV-seropositive patients are predisposing factors acting synergistically with the immune deficiency. Conventional topical treatment is usually adequate.

Iris

Although HIV can cause a primary anterior uveitis, more commonly there is inflammation in the posterior segment.

Retina and choroid

HIV microvasculopathy similar to that involving the conjunctiva can affect the retinal vessels and is extremely common. It is not infective. The most frequent sign is the cotton wool spot; other features include retinal haemorrhages and microaneurysms. Sight is not affected and no therapeutic measure is indicated.

Cytomegalovirus is the organism responsible for a severe retinitis that is very common in patients with advanced AIDS, occurring in about 25%. It represents a considerable threat to vision, with about half of affected patients suffering severe visual loss by the time of death.

Presenting symptoms include blurring and a shimmering effect, but detection may follow routine examination. There is usually no iritis or vitritis. The retinal appearance is said to resemble a pizza, with areas of dense white-yellow

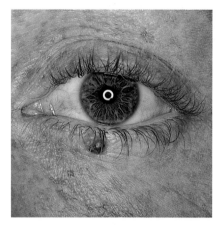

Fig. 1 **Kaposi's sarcoma of the eyelid.**

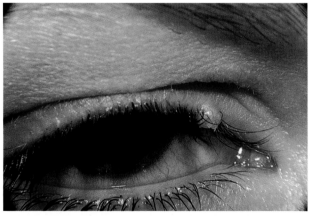

Fig. 2 **Lesion of molluscum contagiosum on eyelid margin.**

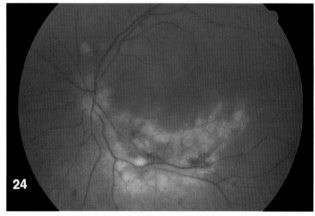

24

Fig. 3 **Cytomegalovirus retinitis.**

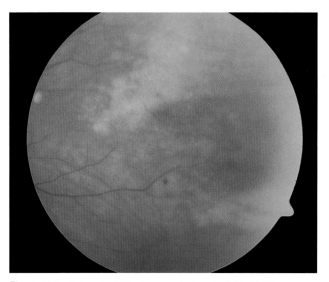

Fig. 4 **Retinal atrophy following regression of CMV retinitis.**

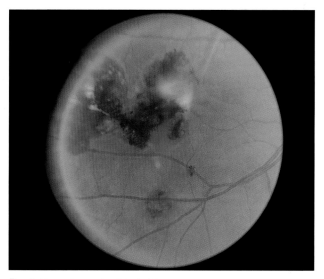

Fig. 5 **Toxoplasmosis with vitritis.**

Table 1 **Treatment of CMV retinitis**		
Drug	**Route**	**Side effects**
Ganciclovir	Intravenous, oral	Pancytopenia, gastrointestinal dysfunction
Ganciclovir	Intravitreal	Complications of method of administration e.g. retinal detachment
Valganciclovir (prodrug of Ganciclovir)	Oral	As ganciclovir
Foscarnet	Intravenous	Nephrotoxicity, seizures, electrolyte imbalance
Cidofovir	Intravenous	Nephrotoxicity, fever, nausea
Note: despite therapy, which must be lifelong, relapses can occur.		

exudate mixed with large flame-shaped haemorrhages (Fig. 3) that spread along retinal vessels. The posterior pole is often preferentially involved. The diagnosis is clinical.

Treatment is with antiviral agents (Table 1).

Although the activity of the retinitis can be curtailed, as the inflammation resolves the necrotic areas become thinned and atrophic (Fig. 4), with a high risk of retinal break formation and consequent retinal detachment. These detachments are very difficult to treat.

Toxoplasma retinochoroiditis is also common in AIDS patients. Whereas in the immunocompetent person reactivation of congenitally acquired latent organisms occurs, in the immunocompromised patient acquired infection is the cause.

Presentation is with blurred vision and floaters. Typical signs of iridocyclitis are common. Vitritis is prominent (in contrast with CMV retinitis). White foci of retinochoroiditis are seen (Fig. 5).

Ocular involvement can be associated with coexistent central nervous system toxoplasmosis in patients with AIDS.

Treatment is with the appropriate oral antibiotics. In contrast to immunocompetent patients with toxoplasmosis, systemic steroids are unnecessary.

A variety of other infectious, largely opportunistic, causes of posterior segment inflammation are more frequent and more severe in patients with HIV. These include **tuberculosis, syphilis, fungal infections** such as candida and cryptococcus and protozoa such as *Pneumocystis carinii*. Herpes viruses can give rise to the **progressive outer retinal necrosis (PORN)** syndrome, in which there is rapidly progressive retinal necrosis with subsequent retinal detachment.

Ocular motility
Abnormalities of eye movement are caused by cranial nerve palsies, brainstem syndromes and cortical disease. Causes include central nervous system lymphoma, and encephalitis and meningitis from opportunistic infections such as toxoplasmosis, mycobacteria, syphilis and a variety of viruses and fungi.

Elevated intracranial pressure from any cause may give rise to a sixth cranial nerve palsy.

Optic nerve
The optic nerve can be affected directly by a range of diseases similar to that affecting the CNS. Optic disc swelling and optic atrophy may be secondary to intraocular disease or elevated intracranial pressure.

Chronic meningeal infection with the fungus *Cryptococcus neoformans* leads to impairment of cerebrospinal fluid absorption and consequently raised intracranial pressure.

Orbit
Orbital non-Hodgkin's lymphoma is not uncommon in patients with AIDS. It causes increasing proptosis which may be painful. Treatment is with local radiotherapy and systemic chemotherapy.

HIV and the eye

- Ocular features may be the first evidence of HIV infection.
- Lids: Kaposi's sarcoma, herpes simplex, herpes zoster ophthalmicus, molluscum contagiosum.
- Conjunctiva/cornea: conjunctival microvasculopathy, Kaposi's sarcoma, dry eye, infection.
- Retina/choroid: retinal microvasculopathy (cotton wool spots), CMV retinitis (commonest severe visual threat), PORN toxoplasma retinochoroiditis, other opportunistic infections.
- Ocular motility disturbance: generally CNS disease.
- Orbit: lymphoma.

Tropical ophthalmology

Many blinding ocular diseases are confined to or are considerably more common in tropical and subtropical regions. The fact that these areas are often also very poor increases the clinical problems, since access to effective treatments and preventative measures is limited (Table 1).

Cataract

Untreated cataract, responsible for approximately half of all blindness, is the most important cause of visual morbidity worldwide.

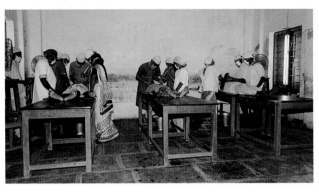

Fig. 1 **An 'eye camp' operating theatre in India.**

Treatment and prevention

The treatment of cataract in developing countries is hindered principally by lack of resources, including a lack of trained personnel. Surgical equipment and operative techniques are frequently rudimentary. In many regions intraocular lens implantation is not possible. Non-prescription aphakic glasses are provided but when these are lost or broken blindness returns. Postoperative review is often very limited and complications may go untreated.

Simple but effective organisational measures, such as the 'eye camp', bring ophthalmic services to the underdeveloped regions (Fig. 1).

Trachoma

Trachoma is a severe form of conjunctivitis caused by infection with *Chlamydia trachomatis*. It is responsible for more blindness on a worldwide basis than any other pathology except cataract. Trachoma is discussed in detail elsewhere (see p. 34).

Xerophthalmia

Vitamin A is essential for the maintenance of the body's epithelial surfaces, for immune function and for the synthesis of retinal photoreceptor proteins. The clinical syndrome of vitamin A deficiency (xerophthalmia) consists of ocular features together with less well-defined systemic characteristics such as a heightened vulnerability to infection. It is the most important cause of blindness amongst children in regions where dietary intake is insufficient for childhood metabolic demands.

Ocular manifestations include night blindness, corneal and conjunctival xerosis (dryness) and keratinisation, silvery-white collections of debris (Bitot's spots) which overlie abnormal areas of conjunctiva, and sharply-demarcated sterile corneal ulcers which may progress to perforation.

Table 1 **Confronting Third World blindness**
Cataract
■ Increasing the availability of surgery
■ Long-term correction of aphakia
Trachoma
■ Improving personal hygiene
Vitamin A deficiency
■ Providing adequate diet and oral supplementation
Onchocerciasis
■ Protecting against the black fly vector
Glaucoma
■ Increasing the availability and affordability of medical treatment

Table 2 **Ocular involvement in vitamin A deficiency**
Night blindness
Cornea
■ Punctate epithelial erosions
■ Sterile ulceration
■ Dryness (xerosis)
■ Keratinisation
■ Bacterial infection
■ Progressive thinning
Conjunctiva
■ Dryness (xerosis)
■ Keratinisation
■ Bitot's spots

Secondary bacterial corneal infection is common. Progressive corneal necrosis (keratomalacia) may occur in advanced xerophthalmia (Table 2).

The diagnosis can be confirmed by conjunctival cytological studies or blood testing.

Treatment and prevention

Definitive treatment is with oral vitamin A. Copious ocular lubrication is also essential initially. Sterile xerophthalmic ulcers will heal with vitamin A replenishment, but specific antibacterial treatment is necessary for infective keratitis. Severe corneal disease can be extremely difficult to treat.

Prevention of xerophthalmia requires a diet rich in vitamin A. In its fat-soluble form the vitamin is found in dairy products, eggs and fish liver oils, and in the provitamin A form in many types of fruit and vegetables. Regular prophylactic supplementation is advocated for susceptible populations.

Onchocerciasis

Onchocerciasis ('river blindness') is caused by infestation with the helminth *Onchocerca volvulus*. Endemic areas are found in equatorial Africa and Central and South America. The disease predominantly involves the skin and eyes, with blindness a common complication.

The vector is the blackfly (*Simulium* family), which breeds around well-oxygenated swift-flowing water. During an incubation period of about a year, a subcutaneous nodule or onchocercoma forms at the location of a blackfly bite, from where an adult female worm sheds microfilariae which migrate through the skin (Fig. 2). Degenerating microfilariae excite a hypersensitivity reaction which accounts for the clinical manifestations of the disease.

A papular rash, pruritus, lichenification and skin thickening may occur. With progression, areas of skin become inelastic and hang in thickened folds.

Eye involvement occurs with severe chronic infestation. Microfilariae probably reach the eye mainly via the conjunctiva. Ocular features include lid nodules and depigmentation, chronic conjunctivitis, a 'snowflake' punctate keratitis, sclerosing keratitis with corneal opacification, chronic iritis with secondary cataract and glaucoma, chorioretinitis and optic neuritis. Microfilariae may be visible on slit lamp examination in the anterior chamber and cornea and are also seen in skin snips. A peripheral blood count will show eosinophilia.

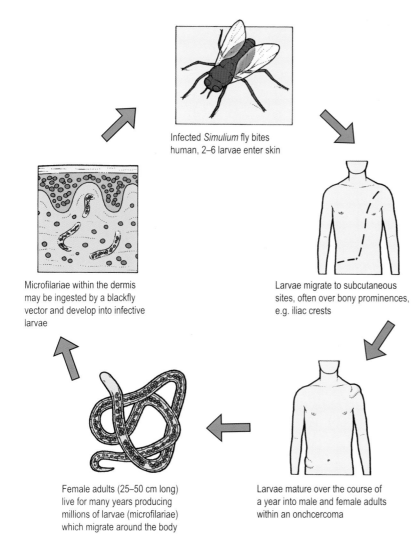

Infected *Simulium* fly bites
human, 2–6 larvae enter skin

Microfilariae within the dermis
may be ingested by a blackfly
vector and develop into infective
larvae

Larvae migrate to subcutaneous
sites, often over bony prominences,
e.g. iliac crests

Female adults (25–50 cm long)
live for many years producing
millions of larvae (microfilariae)
which migrate around the body

Larvae mature over the course of
a year into male and female adults
within an onchcercoma

Fig. 2 **Cycle of *Onchocerca volvolus* infection.**

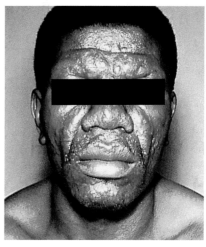

Fig. 3 **Facial appearance of a patient with lepromatous leprosy.** (Courtesy D.J. Gawkrodger.)

Table 3 **Blindness in leprosy**
Corneal exposure
Corneal anaesthesia
Dry eyes
Cataract and glaucoma due to iritis

Treatment and prevention

Treatment with ivermectin will effectively and safely reduce microfilarial numbers though a cure is not achieved. Ivermectin is given as a single dose once a year. In endemic areas the entire population is treated. Measures to reduce the transmission of infection centre around the blackfly vector and range from simple personal protection to habitat eradication.

Leprosy

Though the prevalence is falling, this slowly progressive granulomatous condition still affects millions in Africa, Southern Asia and elsewhere. *Mycobacterium leprae*, the causative microorganism, is acquired in childhood by contact with infected nasal secretions.

The skin, peripheral nerves and the eyes are the principal sites of clinical involvement. Leprosy can be classified into two forms, tuberculoid and lepromatous. Tuberculoid patients develop discrete hypopigmented anaesthetic skin patches, often on one part of the body such as a limb or the face, together with thickening of isolated peripheral nerves. Histologically, lesions resemble the granulomata of tuberculosis. In the lepromatous variant, there is impairment of cell-mediated immunity. Features are more extensive and progressive with less well-defined areas of skin and nerve infiltration. Marked facial deformity frequently results (Fig. 3). Mucous membrane involvement, nerve palsies and atrophy of the peripheries may all occur. The histology differs from the tuberculoid form and, in particular, bacilli are more evident (Ziehl–Neelsen stain).

The eyes are involved in up to 90% of patients and approximately 20% of late-stage patients may be blind (Table 3).

A particular problem associated with the blindness of leprosy is the coexistent peripheral anaesthesia, which significantly compounds the handicap.

Eyebrow and eyelash loss may be seen. The inadequate eyelid closure and ectropion of a facial nerve palsy can lead to corneal exposure and ulceration, often worsened by corneal anaesthesia and dry eyes. Inflammatory manifestations include keratitis, episcleritis, scleritis and acute and chronic iritis. 'Iris pearls', tiny whitish formations consisting of bacilli and inflammatory cells, may develop on the iris surface.

Treatment and prevention

Systemic treatment with dapsone, rifampicin and clofazimine ('multidrug therapy') is frequently required for years.

Much specific ocular management is simple and cheap, such as education about regular active blinking and basic hygiene. The application of topical lubricant preparations is likely to be necessary. Iritis and its complications are managed as appropriate, and abnormalities of the eyelids can often be effectively treated surgically.

Tropical ophthalmology

- Management of treatable ophthalmic disease is hindered by poverty.
- Cataract is the major cause of blindness.
- Infectious causes of blindness (trachoma, onchocerciasis, leprosy) remain important.
- Vitamin A deficiency may lead to the clinical syndrome of xerophthalmia, particularly in childhood.

Epidemiology and the functional implications of visual impairment

Visual impairment is the most obviously disabling consequence of eye disease. Severe loss of sight has major functional and social implications, inevitably resulting in considerable handicap.

Epidemiology

The prevalence of visual impairment is extremely difficult to establish. In general, visual morbidity is under-reported. Only 1 in 3 of the population and 1 in 10 of those over the age of 75 who are eligible for blind or partial sight registration are actually registered.

In Western countries, the prevalence of blindness is probably around 0.2%. The conditions commonly responsible are associated with ageing and include macular degeneration (50%) and glaucoma (10%). Diabetic retinopathy accounts for 3%, and a miscellaneous variety of inherited and acquired conditions accounts for 30%. About 20% of registered cases are for diseases which may be preventable if treated effectively.

The prevalence of blindness is much higher in developing countries, and in the least developed may be 3% or more. The frequency of blindness among children in particular is considerably higher than in the developed world. Many millions of people in poorer countries are blind from treatable cataract. Infections such as trachoma and onchocerciasis are far more common, with a scarcity of the appropriate treatments and of the sanitary conditions necessary for their prevention. Inadequate nutrition can lead to xerophthalmia, a disease of vitamin A deficiency with severe corneal and retinal complications.

Prevention of blindness

The natural history of many causes of blindness can be modified by early intervention. In developing countries, the detection and treatment of a variety of important conditions such as cataract and infectious disease are relatively straightforward. Lack of resources is the major obstacle to a substantial reduction in morbidity.

In many developed countries, screening programmes for diabetic retinopathy (Fig. 1) have been developed, since it is a common treatable disease causing significant morbidity in an easily identifiable at-risk population. Glaucoma is less suitable, though recent advances in our understanding of the disease and of treatment choices should enable resources to be targeted at 'at risk' individuals.

Definition of blindness: blind registration

The range of severity of visual impairment is broad, extending from the minimal symptoms of early cataract to the total blindness (no perception of light), of advanced glaucoma. Though a layman might not consider the person with vision of 3/60 as truly blind, the performance of any task requiring visual guidance, including many vocational activities, is obviously severely hampered at this level of vision. The extent of handicap due to blindness is dependent on factors other than just measured acuity, such as the pattern of visual field defect (Fig. 2), the patient's age at the time of sight loss, individual motivation and the presence of any coexisting physical disability.

In the UK, the formulation of a legal definition of blindness is an attempt to provide an objective standard according to which social support can be targeted (Table 1) and to facilitate the collection of epidemiological data. A register of blind and partially sighted people living in a district is maintained by the local social services department, and addition to this constitutes 'registration'. The process of

Table 1 **Benefits of registration (UK)**
■ Free directory enquiry telephone calls
■ Disabled person's railcard
■ Free postage for specially adapted or designed items
■ Special income tax allowance (blind registration only)
■ Free sight testing
■ Home care and adaptations to the home
■ Training to cope with daily activities and to get about safely
■ Tape and library services

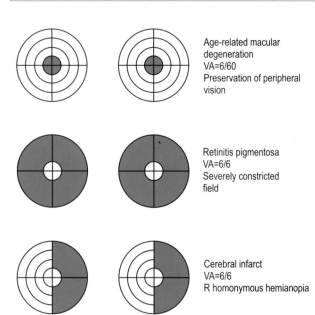

Age-related macular degeneration
VA=6/60
Preservation of peripheral vision

Retinitis pigmentosa
VA=6/6
Severely constricted field

Cerebral infarct
VA=6/6
R homonymous hemianopia

Fig. 2 **Common patterns of 'blinding' field loss.**

Fig. 1 **Mobile screening for diabetic retinopathy.** Unit includes retinal camera. Photographs are examined at base.

Table 2 Guidelines for certification as visually impaired (United Kingdom)*

Best corrected visual acuity	Visual field	Eligibility
<3/60	Irrelevant when acuity is this poor	Blind
>3/60, <6/60	Significantly constricted	Blind
>6/60	Severely constricted, especially inferiorly	Blind
>3/60, <6/60	Full	Partially sighted
<6/18, >6/60	Significantly constricted	Partially sighted
>6/18	Severe constriction or defect (e.g. homonymous hemianopia)	Partially sighted

Note: < worse than; > better than; * some flexibility is possible when considering partial sight certification, but should only rarely be applied to certification as blind

certification as 'legally partially sighted' or 'blind' may only be performed by a senior ophthalmologist (Table 2). A patient is eligible for registration as blind when the best corrected vision is less than 3/60. Substantial visual field defects are taken into account and can lead to registration at better levels of Snellen acuity. The criteria for partial sight registration are more flexible, suggesting eligibility with visual acuity of better than 3/60 but worse than 6/60. As with blind registration, any visual field defect is considered.

Special recommendations apply with regard to the registration of young children.

Community support (Table 3)

Following registration, the social services department carries out a thorough assessment of the patient's home environment to identify practical requirements. Advice, counselling and support are also provided regarding other areas, such as employment, education and leisure activities. Many social services departments employ a rehabilitation officer specialising in the needs of the visually handicapped.

Services for the visually impaired are also provided by voluntary organisations, to whom work may be contracted

out by public authorities. These groups are frequently able to offer access to technical resources, a variety of social facilities and events, impartial advice and practical help.

A range of state financial benefits is available to registered persons.

Low vision aids

When vision is inadequate for the completion of routine tasks despite best refractive correction using spectacles or contact lenses, supplementary devices or 'low vision aids' can often increase the effectiveness of residual function. Most low vision aids assist near-work, especially reading. Examples (Fig. 3) include simple convex magnifying lenses, telescopes and closed-circuit television devices. Many books are available in large print format. Adequate, directed lighting is essential.

Driving regulations

The following information relates to the legal standards applicable in the United Kingdom (Table 4).

The driver of a private car must be able to read a licence plate consisting of letters 79.4 mm high at a distance of 20.5 m, with spectacle or contact lens correction if required. This equates to a Snellen chart level of between 6/9 and 6/12. The minimum acceptable binocular visual field to a specified stimulus intensity extends horizontally for 120 degrees and vertically 20 degrees above and below the horizontal meridian.

The regulations for eligibility to drive a passenger-carrying vehicle (PCV, e.g. a coach), or a large goods vehicle (LGV) are more stringent. The unaided acuity must be better than 3/60 in either eye (monocularity is not permitted), with corrected levels of at least 6/9 in the better eye and 6/12 in the worse eye. The presence of any visual field defect is a bar to driving a PCV or LGV.

Uncorrected diplopia is also a bar to driving any vehicle.

Table 3 Sources of information and advice in UK

Local social services
Local education authority
Local society for visually impaired people
RNIB (020 7388 1266; www.rnib.org.uk)
Department of Health helpline 0800-665544

Table 4 Driving regulations (UK)

Category of vehicle	Minimum visual acuity	Binocular visual field	Diplopia
Private car	Between 6/9 and 6/12 in best eye Monocularity permitted	120 degrees horizontally plus 20 degrees above and below the horizontal meridian (to a specified stimulus)*	Permitted if controlled by prisms or occlusion
Large goods vehicle (LGV) and passenger carrying vehicle (PCV)	Uncorrected: 3/60 in each eye Corrected: 6/9 in best eye, 6/12 in worst eye Monocularity not permitted	Field defect not permitted	Not permitted

*a degree of flexibility may be allowed.

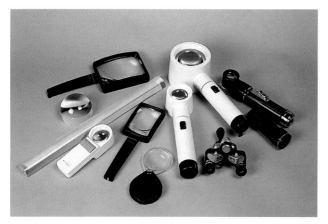

Fig. 3 **Selection of low vision aids.**

> ### *Epidemiology and the functional implications of visual impairment*
>
> - Epidemiology: in developed countries, common causes of blindness are associated with ageing; elsewhere, infections, untreated cataract and childhood blindness are more prevalent.
>
> - Registration as 'legally' blind or partially sighted facilitates social support and epidemiological data collection.
>
> - Social support: social services department, voluntary organisations, financial benefits.
>
> - Low vision aids: typically optimise use of remaining near vision; convex lenses, telescopes, closed-circuit television.
>
> - Driving standards: minimum visual acuity and field are specified; differ for private cars and goods/passenger vehicles.

Ophthalmic surgery

The most common surgical procedures are cataract extraction, retinal detachment repair, glaucoma drainage and correction of strabismus and eyelid abnormalities.

Anaesthesia

The chief goal of the administration of anaesthetic is the prevention of pain, which may be achieved by local or general anaesthetic. An increasingly large proportion of operations are undertaken using local anaesthetic, with general anaesthetic reserved for the uncooperative or very anxious adult patient and for children.

Local anaesthesia

The minimum anaesthetic is a rapidly acting drop such as oxybuprocaine (benoxinate) or tetracaine (amethocaine). Even cataract surgery can be performed with this minimalist approach, but more often an injection technique is used. The favoured agent is lidocaine, with or without adrenaline. Bupivacaine is longer acting and so is often added.

Ocular analgesia and akinesia are achieved by retrobulbar, or peribulbar sub-Tenon's injection (Fig. 1). In the former, the needle is passed into the space behind the globe formed by the rectus muscles. It is very effective, but hazardous. Chief complications are retrobulbar haemorrhage and perforation of the eyeball. Peribulbar injection is safer. The needle is introduced into the soft tissues of the orbit around the globe and the rectus muscle cone. However, the time to onset of effect is longer. In sub-Tenon's injection, a blunt curved cannula is passed along the surface of the eyeball to the retrobulbar space.

Cataract surgery

Improvements in techniques of cataract removal and correction of the resultant refractive error by the insertion of an intraocular lens implant rank amongst the major medical advances of the last twenty years (Table 1). This success is due to several factors including the use of the surgical microscope and an understanding of the need to protect the corneal endothelium. Sadly, cataract is still the major cause of blindness worldwide.

Modern cataract surgery involves removal of the cataract using a probe inserted through a small incision (Fig. 2) and insertion of a folded intraocular lens (IOL or implant) (Fig. 3). A transparent viscoelastic substance made of hyaluronic acid is first injected into the anterior chamber, providing the corneal endothelium with a protective layer. A disc of anterior capsule is peeled off the lens, affording access to the lens nucleus and cortex. The probe mechanically breaks up the lens nucleus into small particles (phacoemulsification), which are sucked out of the eye. A constant flow of saline cools the tip of the probe and helps to maintain the anterior chamber depth. After removal of the nucleus, residual cortex must be aspirated from the eye. The implant is placed within the capsular bag.

The chief peroperative complication is breakage of the capsular bag, usually leading to anterior movement of vitreous gel and sometimes to retention of nuclear fragments in the vitreous cavity. These must be removed by a vitrectomy technique. Postoperative intraocular infection (endophthalmitis) is a rare but devastating complication; the most common late complication is opacification of the capsular bag, treated by laser capsulotomy.

Demographic changes mean that larger numbers of cataract operations are now required. Small incision cataract surgery can be performed rapidly allowing the organisation of 'high volume' operating lists with short turnaround times. Since complication rates are low and visual results high, the visual acuity level at which cataract removal is performed has fallen. For the patient, recovery and stabilisation of vision is rapid. However, the equipment, instrumentation and implant are expensive.

Failure to achieve good vision postoperatively is usually due to pre-existing disease, rather than surgical failure. Amblyopia and macular disease (age-related degeneration and diabetic maculopathy) are important causes.

Intraocular lenses

Rigid PMMA, a form of plastic, has been available for many years and is known to be safe and well tolerated by the eye.

Small incision cataract surgery has stimulated the development of a variety of implants which can be folded for insertion into the eye and which then unfold when correctly

Table 1	**Success and complications of cataract surgery**
Benefits	Improved quality of life
	80–90% achieve 6/12 vision or better
Peroperative complications	Expulsive haemorrhage
	Rupture of posterior capsule with vitreous loss
Postoperative complications	Intraocular infection (endophthalmitis)
	Corneal astigmatism
	Opacification of posterior capsule (treatment = laser capsulotomy)
	Macular oedema
	Retinal detachment

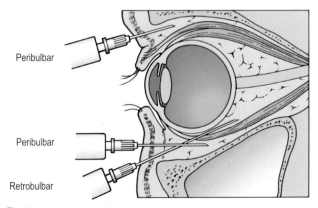

Peribulbar

Peribulbar

Retrobulbar

Fig. 1 **Retrobulbar and peribulbar anaesthesia.**

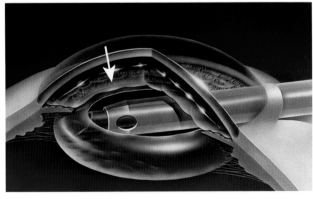

Fig. 2 **Cataract surgery by phacoemulsification: a probe removes lens material from within the capsular bag. A layer of viscoelastic (arrowed) coats and protects the corneal endothelium.**

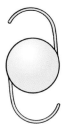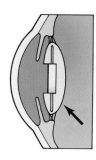

The posterior chamber lens implant
is placed in the capsular bag (arrow)

Fig. 3 **Posterior chamber intraocular lens implant.**

located. Materials include silicone, hydrogel and acrylic.

The postoperative refractive power of the eye depends upon the refractive power of the implant, so choice of an implant of appropriate strength is critical for optimum vision. The implant required to achieve a given post-operative refraction can be predicted from measurement of corneal curvature (keratometry) and the length of the eyeball (measured by ultrasound).

It is usual to render the eye normally sighted (emmetropic), having good unaided distance vision but requiring reading glasses.

Strabismus surgery

Most cases of strabismus are horizontal deviations (convergent or divergent) and can be corrected by weakening and strengthening procedures on the medial and lateral recti (Fig. 4). An analogy may be made with horse-riding: if you wish the horse to turn left, you let out the right rein (weakening procedure) and pull on the left rein (strengthening procedure).

Since we have two eyes and since correct alignment is relative to the other eye, combinations of these procedures can be used to achieve the desired effect.

The main postoperative problem is failure to achieve perfect alignment, which is especially likely in large deviations and in the absence of binocular vision. Therefore, in adults, it is common to employ an adjustable technique. Under general anaesthesia, one muscle is sutured with a bow instead of a knot. Later, with the patient awake, the bow is undone so that the eye position can be adjusted. The suture is then tied to secure it.

Other types of strabismus may require surgery to the vertically-acting muscles. The principles are similar, but it is more difficult to achieve perfect alignment.

Retinal detachment

Most cases of retinal detachment (see page 64) are due to a tear in the retina caused by traction exerted by attached vitreous. Fluid passes from the vitreous into the subretinal space and the retina detaches. Surgery involves relief of traction, by removal of vitreous (vitrectomy) or by indentation of the globe using a piece of silicone (an 'explant') sutured to the sclera, and creation of a chorioretinal adhesion, by laser or cryotherapy.

Often the subretinal fluid is drained to help retinal reattachment, and the retinal tear occluded by injection of gas or air.

Surgery usually results in re-attachment, but central vision is permanently impaired if the macula has been detached for more than a few days. Proliferation of scar tissue on the surface of the retina, leading to redetachment, is the main complication.

Glaucoma

Most cases of glaucoma are caused by failure of normal aqueous outflow through the trabecular meshwork. Surgery (trabeculectomy) involves the creation of a new outflow channel, draining into a space under the conjunctiva (see page 45).

The chief complications are acceleration of cataract and occlusive fibrosis of the new channel, which is particularly likely to occur in certain types of glaucoma. Peroperative application of an antiproliferative drug such as 5-fluorouracil can reduce the incidence of failure.

Trabeculectomy is often combined with cataract extraction.

Corneal transplantation

The main reason for full-thickness removal of the cornea and its replacement with donor material is opacity, typically the result of scarring, a dystrophy or endothelial failure.

Donor eyes can be removed post mortem and the cornea stored in a special medium for up to 30 days. Tissue typing is not necessary, and rejection is less frequent than for other organs, so topical immunosuppression alone (steroid drops) is usual.

Visual success is often limited by graft astigmatism. Preoperative vascularisation of the host cornea increases the risk of rejection. Herpetic keratitis or dystrophy may recur in the graft.

Refractive surgery

Surgery for myopia, hypermetropia and astigmatism is in increasing demand and is a rapidly developing field. Further details are found on page 85.

Surgery to the eyelids

Removal of a variety of small lesions can be achieved without difficulty and with good cosmesis, particularly because facial skin has great reparative powers. Excision of larger lesions and repair of the resultant defect requires special training, as eyelid reconstruction must achieve cosmesis and adequate protection of the globe without corneal exposure.

Positional deformities of the lower lid (entropion and ectropion) are common. Ptosis is more difficult to treat, since correction can be excessive, leading to corneal exposure.

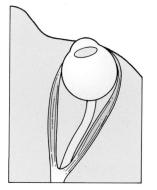

Right eye is convergent

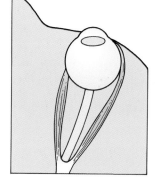

Lateral rectus is resected
Medial rectus is recessed

Fig. 4 **Horizontal rectus weakening and strengthening operations.**

Ophthalmic surgery

- Anaesthesia:
  – local anaesthesia by sub-Tenon's retro- and peribulbar injection is very effective
  – chief complications of local anaesthesia are orbital haemorrhage and ocular perforation.

- Cataract surgery:
  – small incision surgery using phacoemulsification and insertion of foldable lens achieves best result
  – poor postoperative vision usually due to pre-existing disease.

- Strabismus surgery:
  – weaken muscle action by recession of insertion
  – enhance muscle action by resection of a segment.

Lasers in ophthalmology

Lasers are used in the management of many ophthalmic conditions, particularly because so many ocular structures can be easily visualised and because of the precision of laser delivery.

Laser instruments are expensive to buy, and it is usual to require more than one type of laser in routine ophthalmic practice.

Stringent safety regulations must be applied because of the risk of laser damage to the eyes of the patient, the operator and any bystander.

The physics of lasers

LASER is an acronym for Light Amplification by Stimulated Emission of Radiation. Energy is applied to a potential light source such as a gas. The applied energy excites atoms, raising their electrons to a higher energy level. When an electron falls back to the lower energy level, it emits a photon of light. In a laser instrument, the process of excitation and photon release is controlled and synchronised so that an extremely bright light is emitted in which the photons are of identical wavelength, are in phase (at the same stage in the wave cycle at any given point) and travel in parallel (Fig. 1).

Types of laser in clinical use

A range of clinical lasers is available (Table 1). The chief difference between them is the material from which the laser light is produced since the material determines the wavelength of light and its mode of action.

Clinical applications

Most laser treatments are performed as out-patient procedures under topical anaesthesia. Rarely a retrobulbar injection is administered to improve pain control or to immobilise the eye completely. Most procedures require or are enhanced by the use of a specialised contact lens, to optimise visualisation of the target tissue, to part the eyelids and to reduce ocular movement.

Some of the diseases amenable to laser treatment were untreatable before the introduction of lasers, and some could only be managed by intraocular surgery, which carries significantly higher risks.

Glaucoma

Laser iridotomy is the treatment of choice for acute angle closure glaucoma caused by pupil block. The iridotomy, placed in the peripheral iris (Fig. 2), allows aqueous humour to pass from the posterior chamber into the anterior chamber without passing through the pupil.

Intraocular pressure control in open angle glaucoma may be improved by argon laser trabeculoplasty, in which a series of laser burns is applied to the trabecular meshwork. The mechanism of action of this procedure is not understood. It is now less popular than when first introduced.

In advanced glaucoma that has been resistant to conventional treatments, destruction of the ciliary body to reduce aqueous humour production can be achieved with the diode and Nd-YAG lasers fired through the sclera.

Several attempts have been made to mimic the action of drainage surgery (trabeculectomy) with lasers, but comparable success has not yet been achieved.

Rubeotic glaucoma, in which iris neovascularisation leads to occlusion of the anterior chamber angle, occurs in response to ocular ischaemia, particularly diabetic retinopathy and retinal vein occlusion. Treatment of the retinal disease with laser may improve the glaucoma.

Posterior capsule opacification

Posterior capsule (PC) thickening, also known as 'after-cataract', is a common late complication of cataract extraction. It occurs as a result of proliferation and metaplasia of residual lens fibres attached to the capsule. Symptoms include poor vision and glare.

Table 1 **Major applications of lasers in ophthalmology**

Type of laser	Major uses	Mode of action
Argon and krypton	Diabetic maculopathy Panretinal photocoagulation for retinal and iris neovascularisation Retinal breaks with or without retinal detachment Destruction of choroidal neovascular membrane in age-related macular degeneration Laser trabeculoplasty (LTP or ALT) Ablation of aberrant eyelashes	Pigments of eye absorb photons and release heat
Nd-YAG[a]	Posterior capsulotomy for 'after-cataract' Peripheral iridotomy	Causes localised tissue disintegration
Excimer	Corneal sculpting for correction of refractive error Treatment of superficial corneal pathology	Disrupts connections between molecules
Diode	Retinal pathology Trans-scleral application to intraocular tissues Photodynamic therapy	Pigments of eye absorb photons and release heat Activation of injected photosensitive agent releasing cytotonic free radicals

[a] **N**eodymium-**Y**ttrium-**A**luminium-**G**arnet

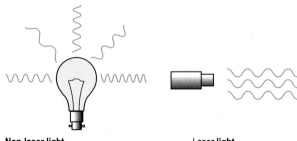

Non-laser light
- random direction
- typically a range of wavelengths
- waves of same length out of phase

Laser light
- parallel
- single or few discrete
- wavelengths
- waves in phase

Fig. 1 **Properties of laser light waves.**

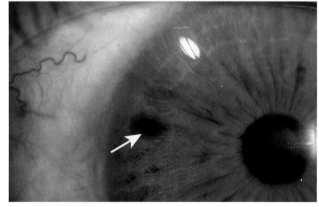

Fig. 2 **Peripheral iridotomy.**

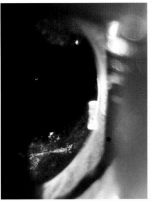
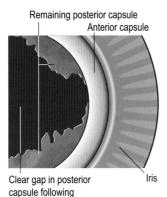

Remaining posterior capsule
Anterior capsule

Clear gap in posterior
capsule following
laser disruption

Iris

Fig. 3 **Posterior capsulotomy.**

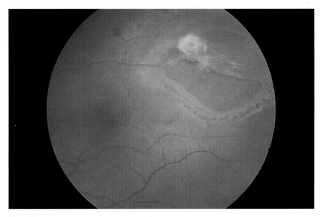

Fig. 5 **Retinal tear surrounded by laser burns.**

The Nd-YAG laser is used to create a central defect in the posterior capsule (Fig. 3). This does not affect the position or integrity of an intraocular lens implant.

There are risks to this laser treatment, including retinal detachment and cystoid macular oedema, so only significant opacification is lasered.

Diabetic retinopathy

Laser treatment of diabetic proliferative retinopathy and macular oedema (see p. 52) has revolutionised the prognosis of these diseases.

In **proliferative diabetic retinopathy**, ischaemic retina stimulates the growth of abnormal 'new vessels', which can bleed and cause retinal detachment. Argon or diode laser treatment of the ischaemic areas (panretinal photocoagulation) causes regression of neovascularisation. The macular area is preserved to maintain central vision (Fig. 4).

Effective treatment significantly reduces the risk of visual loss from proliferative diabetic retinopathy. However, extensive laser application can constrict the visual field and may exacerbate macular oedema.

The role of panretinal photocoagulation in **pre-proliferative retinopathy** has not yet been established, but most specialists would treat severe disease to prevent progression to the proliferative stage.

During intraocular surgery for **diabetic tractional retinal detachment**, laser may be applied directly to the retina.

Certain types of **diabetic macular oedema** respond to gentle argon laser treatment, but the mechanism is unclear and there is a risk of inadvertent foveal damage causing permanent reduction in vision and impairment of colour discrimination.

Laser is also of some benefit in the macular oedema and retinal neovascularisation which occurs in subgroups of retinal vein occlusion.

Age-related macular degeneration

Growth of a choroidal neovascular membrane (CNVM) ('wet' ARMD) causes rapidly progressive sight loss. In photodynamic therapy (PDT) (see p. 59), a photosensitive agent injected intravenously is taken up by the CNVM and activated by application of a nonthermal laser, resulting in destruction of the membrane. However, few patients are suitable and visual outcome depends on the health of the overlying retina.

Laser has no role in the management of the more common 'dry' form of macular degeneration.

Retinal detachment

A retinal tear or hole without retinal detachment can be surrounded with laser to induce adhesion and prevent retinal detachment (Fig. 5). During retinal detachment surgery, laser is sometimes used as an alternative to cryotherapy to promote retinal adhesion.

Refractive errors

The excimer laser, applied with computer assistance, very precisely removes corneal tissue in the management of myopia, hypermetropia and astigmatism.

Miscellaneous uses

- Ablation of intraocular and adnexal tumours.
- Division of intraocular postinflammatory adhesions.
- Destruction of aberrant eyelashes.
- Removal of superficial corneal scars and calcific band keratopathy (excimer laser).

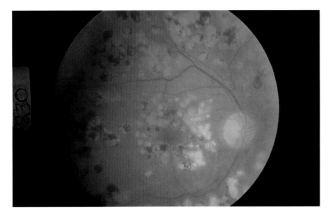

Fig. 4 **Laser scars following panretinal photocoagulation and macular laser.** The fovea has been spared.

> ### Lasers in ophthalmology
>
> - Lasers emit photons of light with a single wavelength that travel in phase and are parallel.
>
> - Glaucoma
>   – Nd-YAG laser peripheral iridotomy in angle closure glaucoma
>   – argon laser trabeculoplasty in open angle glaucoma.
>
> - Posterior capsule opacification treated with Nd-YAG laser.
>
> - Diabetic retinopathy: panretinal photocoagulation for proliferative retinopathy; gentle macular laser for maculopathy.
>
> - Age-related macular degeneration can sometimes be treated by ablation of a choroidal neovascular membrane.
>
> - Laser around retinal breaks can prevent or treat retinal detachment.
>
> - Refractive errors (especially myopia) can be treated with the excimer laser.

Ocular genetics

A clinical approach to ocular genetics

Recognition that an ocular condition has a genetic basis occurs when an alert clinician takes an accurate family history (e.g. glaucoma, cataract) or makes a clinical diagnosis which has a known genetic aetiology (e.g. retinitis pigmentosa – RP). The clinician should then:

- Characterise the ocular findings as completely as possible, in order to:
  - define the phenotype
  - assist in the clinical and genetic diagnosis
  - document disease progression (e.g. RP)
- Define and record non-ocular features
- Take a full history, including consanguinity and fetal loss, and record the family tree (Fig. 1A), which assists in determining the inheritance pattern:
  - autosomal dominant, autosomal recessive, X-linked (Mendelian)
  - mitochondrial
- Examine all available family members, 'affected' and 'unaffected', to determine disease status
- Contact the local clinical ocular genetics service:

- assistance in characterising the disorder
- coordinate referral to other medical specialties
- for genetic counselling
- mutational screening and genetic diagnosis
- Access information sources to aid diagnosis:
  - NCBI Entrez:
    http://www.ncbi.nlm.nih.gov/entrez/
  - Pubmed:
    http://www.ncbi.nlm.nih.gov/PubMed
  - Online Mendelian Inheritance in Man (OMIM):
    http://www.ncbi.nlm.nih.gov/entrez/ query.fcgi?db=OMIM
  - RetNet:
    http://www.sph.uth.tmc.edu/Retnet/
  - LensNet Human Lens Genetic Disease Database:
    http://ken.mitton.com/ern/ lensbase.html

The ophthalmologist's role in defining the clinical phenotype is central to subsequent genetic diagnosis and the quality of input from the clinical genetic service. Making a genetic diagnosis remains challenging as the identification of genes and genetic defects causing ocular disease

continually increases. Written information can become obsolete quickly and the internet is a vital resource to access current data about phenotype and disease genes, and provides search tools integrated with the literature and genetic data (Entrez, PubMed, OMIM).

Finding disease genes

In a family with inherited eye disease
Having identified a family with a genetic eye disease and documented the mode of inheritance and the disease status of all available family members, the next step is to find the disease-causing gene. One approach is to select candidate loci or genes, on the basis of known gene mutations or genetic linkage studies that produce similar ocular phenotypes, for haplotype and linkage analysis (Fig. 2). The family is typed with genetic markers. Markers which are closely linked to the disease-causing gene are usually inherited together more often than chance alone. This relationship is statistically described by the LOD score (logarithm of odds): a ratio of the likelihood or probability that loci are linked versus the likelihood that they are not linked. A LOD score of 3 supports linkage while a score of -2 excludes linkage.

The LOD score has limited power in smaller families. Haplotype analysis can be used to study smaller families to assess the association of phenotype with a genetic locus. The haplotype is the combination of alleles or marker scores at a specific chromosomal location. Linkage and haplotype analyses can identify likely disease-causing genes which can be then be screened for mutations. Alternatively, if the family is large enough, the whole genome of the individuals can be typed with hundreds of regularly spaced genetic markers – a genome-wide scan.

In an individual with inherited eye disease
Identifying the disease-causing gene in an individual or in a family that is too small for linkage or haplotype analysis can be difficult, time-consuming and expensive. Genetic heterogeneity means that identical phenotypes can be caused

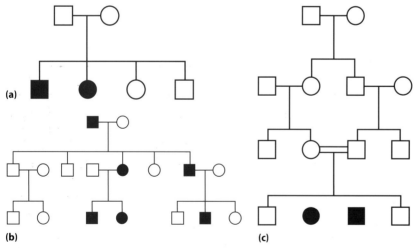

Fig. 1 **Basic Mendelian patterns of inheritance. (a)** Males are represented by squares and females by circles. Blackened symbols indicate clinically affected individuals; unblackened symbols represent unaffected relatives; female gene carriers are represented by circles with black central dots. Consanguineous marriages are represented by double lines connecting pairings. **(b) Autosomal dominant:** affected individuals are directly related through successive generations; affects either sex and is transmitted by either sex; trait does not occur in offspring of unaffected individuals; 50% risk with each pregnancy of child being affected. **(c) Autosomal recessive:** affected individuals are usually born to unaffected parents; unaffected parents are usually asymptomatic carriers; affects either sex; increased incidence of parental consanguinity; the risk of having an affected child is 25%.

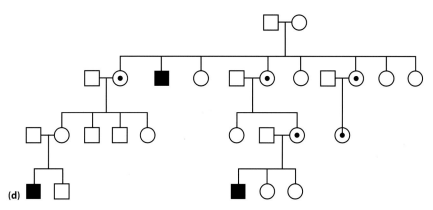

(d)

Fig. 1 **Basic Mendelian patterns of inheritance. (d) X-linked recessive:** affects mainly males; no male-to-male transmission in the family; affected males usually born to unaffected parents with the mother being an asymptomatic carrier who may have affected male relatives; carrier females may show some features of the disorder (e.g. X-linked RP); all the daughters of affected males will be carriers but no son will be affected.

by two or more genes, so that deciding which genes to screen for defects is difficult. A karyotype (chromosomal spread) may be helpful, since on rare occasions an affected individual can have a chromosomal translocation or deletion which disrupts a gene causing the observed phenotype.

A number of techniques with different sensitivity, expense (time and money) and technical difficulty can be used to screen for mutations in a potential disease gene. As mutational screening in ocular genetics becomes more commonplace, the assistance and advice of a clinical geneticist is mandatory in interpreting mutational reports and dealing with potential clinical scenarios. A negative result may mean that the coding sequence change was missed within the technical constraints of the experimental method employed, or that the mutation may be in an intronic regulatory element or upstream promoter, or a different gene is responsible. If a sequence change is detected its pathogenicity must be assessed.

In order to determine whether a detected sequence change is disease-causing, the following are considered:

- Segregation: all affected family members have the mutation whereas unaffected family members do not.
- Controls: ethnically and age-matched normal controls have been screened and do not have the mutation.
- Amino acid sequence: is the biochemistry of a substituted amino acid or protein structure altered?
- Conservation: is the amino acid residue conserved across species suggesting strong evolutionary conservation?
- Gene expression: does the biological expression of the gene make sense when considering the phenotype?
- Functional studies: is there a functional assay which can demonstrate the pathological effects of the sequence change?
- Murine models: genetically engineered mice can confirm the pathogenicity of the genetic defect.

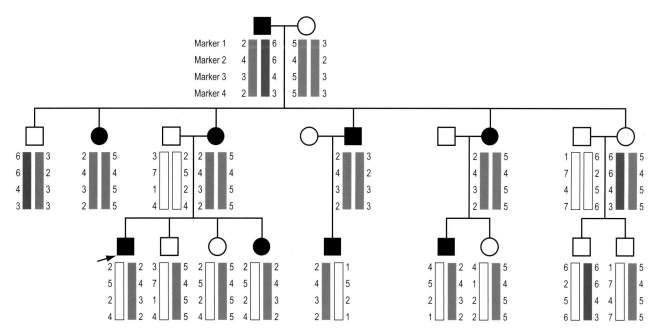

Fig. 2 **Haplotype and linkage analysis.** Hypothetical pedigree with ocular genetic disease showing autosomal dominant inheritance with the proband or index case identified by the arrow. Haplotype analysis shows the segregation of four hypothetical genetic markers (1–4) around a known disease gene. The disease haplotype segregates with the phenotype and is indicated as a red bar with the alleles: Marker 1 (allele 2); Marker 2 (allele 4); Marker 3 (allele 3) and Marker 4 (allele 2). An allele is one of many potential alternative forms of DNA or gene at a specific chromosomal location; here the numbers for each marker indicate which allele form the individual has for that genetic marker. The maximum LOD score was achieved for Marker 1 giving a value of 4.6, confirming linkage of the phenotype to the disease gene associated with markers.

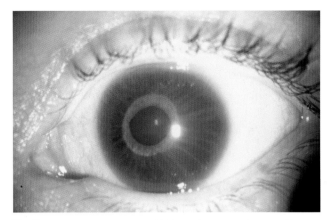

Fig. 3 **Anterior segment view of iridogoniodysgenesis caused by a *FOCX1* mutation.**

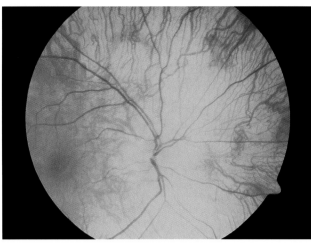

Fig. 4 **Fundal view of choroideraemia caused by a mutation in *CHM* gene.**

Using these approaches a number of genes have been identified that cause ocular disease (Tables 1 and 2). These studies highlight the high degree of genetic heterogeneity among ocular genetic diseases, with many genes responsible for a single clinical entity like retinitis pigmentosa. A number of challenges must be overcome before genetic testing becomes mainstream in clinical practice.

Table 2 The genetic basis of glaucoma

Glaucoma type*	Location	Gene
POAG/JOAG	1q23-25	*TIGR/myocilin*
POAG	2cen-q13	?
POAG	3q21-q24	?
PAOG	8q23	?
POAG (NTG)	10p15-p14	*OPTN*
POAG	7q	?
PCG	2p21 (AR)	*CYP1B1*
PCG	1p36 (AR)	?
Rieger syndrome	4q25	*PITX2*
IGDA	6p25	*FOXC1*
Nail-patella syndrome	9q34	*LMX1B*
Anterior segment dysgenesis	10q25	*PITX3*
Aniridia	11p13	*PAX6*

*POAG: primary open angle glaucoma; JOAG: juvenile open angle glaucoma; NTG: normal tension glaucoma; PCG: primary congenital glaucoma; IGDA: iridogoniodysgenesis anomaly.

Table 1 Illustrative overview of the genetic basis of inherited retinal disease

Gene symbol	Gene name	Phenotype*
RPE 65	retinal pigment epithelium-specific 65 kD protein	LCA (AR); RP (AR)
ABCA4	ATP-binding cassette transporter-retinal	STG (AR); FFM (AR); RP (AR)
CRB1	crumbs homolog 1	LCA (AR); RP (AR)
MERTK	Protein c-mer proto-oncogene receptor tyrosine kinase	RP (AR)
SAG	arrestin (S-antigen)	Oguchi disease (AR); RP (AR)
PDE6A	rod cGMP phosphodiesterase α subunit	RP (AR)
PDE6B	rod cGMP phosphodiesterase β subunit	RP (AR); CSNB (AD)
TULP1	tubby-like protein 1	RP (AR)
RHO	rhodopsin	RP (AD); CSNB (AD)
RDS	peripherin	RP (AD), AVMD (AD); PD (AD)
RP1	RP1 protein	RP (AD)
ROM1	retinal outer segment membrane protein 1	RP (AD)
CRX	cone-rod otx-like photoreceptor homeobox	LCA (AD/AR); RP (AD); CRD (AD)
PRPF31	human homolog of yeast pre-mRNA splicing factor	RP (AD)
RP2	XRP2 protein	RP (XL)
RPGR	retinitis pigmentosa GTPase regulator	RP (XL); CSNB (XL)
RPGRIP1	RPGR-interacting protein 1	LCA (AR)
AIPL1	arylhydrocarbon-interacting receptor protein-like 1	LCA (AR); CRD (AD)
GUCY2D	Retinal specific guanylate cyclase	LCA (AR); CRD (AD)
CNGA3	cone photoreceptor cGMP-gated cation channel α3 subunit	achromatopsia (AR)
CNGB3	cone cyclic nucleotide-gated cation channel β3 subunit	achromatopsia (AR)
RHOK	rhodopsin kinase	CSNB (AR)
CACNA1F	L-type voltage-gated calcium channel α-1 subunit	CSNB (XL)
NYX	nyctalopin	CSBN (XL)
ELOVL4	elongation of very long fatty acids protein	macular dystrophy (AD)
VMD2	bestrophin	Best's dystrophy (AD)
TIMP3	tissue inhibitor of metalloproteinases-3	Sorsby's (AD)
RS1	retinoschisin	retinoschisis (XL)
USH2A	usherin	Usher syndrome (AR)
USH1C	harmonin	Usher syndrome (AR)
MYO7A	myosin VIIA	Usher syndrome (AR)
CHM	Geranylgeranyl transferase Rab escort protein	choroideraemia (XL)

*AD: autosomal dominant; AR: autosomal recessive; XL: X-linked; LCA: Leber's congenital amaurosis; RP: retinitis pigmentosa; STG: Stargardt's disease; FFM: fundus flavimaculatus; CRD: cone-rod dystrophy; AVMD: adult vitelliform macular dystrophy; PD: pattern dystrophy; CSNB: congenital stationary night blindness.

Ocular genetics

- Positive family history and specific ocular features can suggest a genetic basis for disease.

- Typical patterns of inheritance are Mendelian and mitochondrial.

- The worldwide web is an important source of information in a rapidly developing field of research and knowledge.

- Many ocular diseases have been found to have a genetic basis, but there is great genetic and clinical heterogeneity and many genes may be responsible for single disease entity.

Clinical decision-making

Gradual visual loss

A 66-year-old man attended his general practitioner (GP) complaining of a painless gradual fall in vision, worse in the right eye than the left, over the preceding six months. Apart from needing spectacles for close work, he had experienced no eye problems in the past. He was known to be hypertensive, but this was well controlled with diuretic tablets. His GP had advised him to consult his optometrist (ophthalmic optician), who was unable to improve the visual acuity by changing his glasses.

Q1: List the major diagnostic possibilities.

SCENARIO 1

The patient had been experiencing increasing difficulty with vision for both near and distance. Bright light caused severe glare. He had had to stop driving. The optometrist found that the patient was more short-sighted than at a previous examination twelve months ago.

Q2: What is the most likely diagnosis, and why?

Q3: What physical sign is demonstrated here (Fig. 1)? What other simple tests could be performed in a GP's surgery to assess further the nature and severity of the problem?

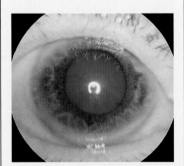

Fig. 1

Q4: What management would you recommend? What is the prognosis?

SCENARIO 2

The patient was beginning to fail to notice objects and people approaching from the side. When crossing the road, he had to turn his head to be sure of seeing approaching traffic.

Q5: What diagnoses would you consider?

Q6: This condition is often initially detected by optometrists. What tests are important in this context?

Q7: These are the patient's optic discs (Fig. 2). Describe what you see.

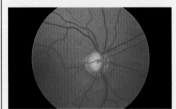

Right

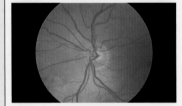

Fig. 2 *Left*

Intraocular pressure was 30 mm Hg in the right eye, and 28 mm Hg in the left. Gonioscopy showed wide open anterior chamber angles in both eyes.

Q8: List the treatment options.

SCENARIO 3

Vision was 6/36 in the right eye, 6/18 in the left. Central vision was reduced, causing considerable difficulty with reading, but peripheral vision was maintained so that navigation and distance vision were less severely affected.

Q9: What is the most likely diagnosis?

Q10: What examination features confirm the diagnosis? What physical signs are seen here (Fig. 3)?

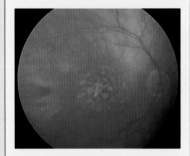

Fig. 3

Q11: What is the management?

A1: The most common causes of gradual visual loss are:

- cataract
- age-related macular degeneration
- diabetic maculopathy
- primary open angle glaucoma.

SCENARIO 1

A2: The most likely diagnosis is cataract. Different morphological types of cataract can cause a variety of symptoms including glare and monocular double vision. Progressive short-sightedness may occur due to a increase in the refractive index of the lens as the cataract becomes more dense.

A3: This is an abnormal red reflex demonstrating a media opacity – in this scenario, cataract. Other simple tests include measurement of the best corrected visual acuity with and without pinhole aperture, the swinging flashlight test to exclude a relative afferent pupil defect and examination of the retina after pupil dilation.

A4: The likely sequel is surgical cataract removal. The decision to operate depends on the severity of the symptoms and the visual demands of the individual. It is likely that a young person will need cataract removal at an earlier stage than an elderly person. Eighty–ninety per cent of operations result in a visual acuity of 6/12 or better. Pre-existing disease, such as macular degeneration, is the main cause of failure to achieve good vision.

SCENARIO 2

A5: The most common cause of gradual loss of peripheral vision is open angle glaucoma. However, patients only experience symptoms when advanced damage is present. Central visual acuity is affected at a very late stage. Other diagnostic possibilities include neurological disease (e.g. homonymous hemianopia) and, uncommonly, unilateral visual loss (cataract etc). Automated visual field analysis for the patient is shown in Figure 4, demonstrating an inferior arcuate scotoma in the right eye.

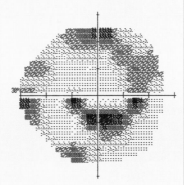

Fig. 4

A6: Measurement of the intraocular pressure, visual field analysis and examination of the optic discs are necessary. A positive family history is an important risk factor for glaucoma, and relatives are advised to undergo regular screening for the disease.

A7: There is advanced cupping of the right optic disc, with a cup/disc ratio of 0.9 and loss of the neuroretinal rim, especially superiorly (consistent with the field loss). The ratio in the left eye is 0.6. The left disc may also be abnormal.

A8: The initial treatment for primary open angle glaucoma is a topical pressure-lowering agent. Provided there is no contraindication, a beta-blocker or prostaglandin analogue is usually first choice. There are several other topical ocular hypotensives which can be used alone or in combination. Laser and surgery are usually withheld until after a trial of medical treatment.

SCENARIO 3

A9: Age-related macular degeneration. Other macular disease, such as diabetic maculopathy, and some forms of cataract can also cause greater difficulty with near rather than distance vision.

A10: Ask the patient to look at your face. Your face will be indistinct, but peripheral vision will be normal to finger testing. Pupil reactions will also be normal. Examination of the macula through dilated pupils may reveal atrophy, pigment clumps and drusen (all illustrated in Fig. 3).

A11: Low vision aids such as hand-held magnifying devices can be very helpful. If vision is sufficiently poor, registration as partially sighted or blind can be arranged. It is important to reassure patients that they will not lose peripheral vision. Other pathology, such as cataract and glaucoma, must be excluded. Sometimes cataract extraction can improve deteriorating navigational vision, but the benefit of surgery is unpredictable.

Gradual visual loss

- Cataract: nuclear sclerosis causes an acquired myopia; glare and reduced vision in bright light occur with other types of opacity; will not cause a relative afferent pupillary defect; examine the red reflex.

- Macular degeneration ('dry' form): reduced central and near vision with preservation of peripheral vision; fundus changes may be subtle.

- Open angle glaucoma: usually asymptomatic until late stage; peripheral vision affected first; examine optic discs.

- Consider diabetic maculopathy due to undiagnosed diabetes mellitus, especially in the elderly.

- Initial referral to an optometrist (ophthalmic optician) for refraction and assessment should be undertaken.

Sudden visual loss

A 75-year-old woman was brought to the ophthalmic emergency clinic by her neighbour. She reported that half an hour previously the vision in her right eye had suddenly been lost. There had been no improvement since. The eye was not painful or red. There was no previous ophthalmic history. Known systemic disease included angina and hypertension, both of which were well controlled with medication.

Q1: What are the chief causes of sudden visual loss?

SCENARIO 1

Vision was 6/60 right, 6/9 left. There was a moderate right relative afferent pupillary defect. The appearance of the retina is shown in Figure 1.

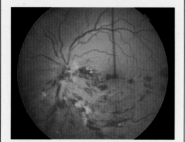

Fig. 1

Q2: What is the diagnosis?

Q3: What systemic investigations are indicated in this patient?

Q4: What are the major ocular complications of this condition?

SCENARIO 2

Vision was 'hand movements' only in the right eye but 6/6 in the left. There was a profound right relative afferent pupillary defect. Ophthalmoscopy of the left eye was normal, but the right optic disc was abnormal (Fig. 2). The right retina was otherwise normal. The remainder of the ocular examination was unremarkable and there was no sign to indicate the presence of an orbital mass.

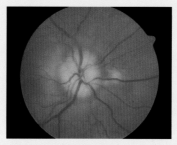

Fig. 2

Q5: What abnormality is shown? What is the likely cause of the visual loss?

On further questioning, the patient reported moderate to severe headaches for the previous six months. She had noticed some tenderness of her scalp whilst brushing her hair. Chewing food caused her jaw to ache. She had felt generally unwell throughout this period and her weight, previously stable, had fallen by five kilos.

Q6: What systemic disease is suggested by this history? What investigations would you request?

Q7: What is the treatment for this condition?

SCENARIO 3

Visual acuities were 6/24 right and 6/6 left. Further questioning revealed that although sight had suddenly deteriorated that day, there had been some distortion for a number of days. The patient described the loss as a constant black patch in the middle of the field of vision of the affected eye. Peripheral vision was preserved (Figs 3 & 4).

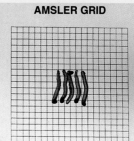

AMSLER GRID

Fig. 3

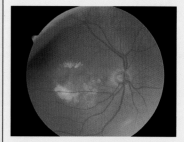

Fig. 4

Q8: What is the likely diagnosis?

Q9: What investigation will assess the macula further?

Q10: The macular lesion was not amenable to treatment. The condition progressed until central vision in the right eye fell to 'counting fingers'. What advice should be given regarding the other eye?

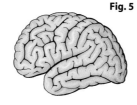

Vitreous
• Vitreous haemorrhage
• retinal detachment

Macula
• age-related macular
  degeneration: exudative type

Optic nerve
• anterior ischaemic optic
  neuropathy: arteritic,
  nonarteritic
• optic neuritis

Fig. 5

Retinal vessels
• retinal venous occlusion: central, branch
• retinal arterial occlusion: central, branch

Cerebral cortex
• stroke: homonymous hemianopia
• sudden awareness of chronic
  monocular loss

A1: Important causes of visual loss of sudden onset in a quiet eye (that is, without significant anterior segment inflammation) are shown in Figure 5. With the exception of optic neuritis, ocular pain is unusual.

SCENARIO 1

A2: This shows a retinal vein occlusion. There are scattered flame-shaped haemorrhages and cotton wool spots, and the optic disc is swollen. The appearance of venous occlusion contrasts greatly with that of central retinal arterial occlusion in which there is a pale oedematous retina, thinned sludged arterioles and a 'cherry red spot' at the fovea (Fig. 6).

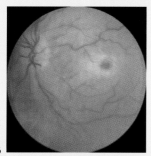

Fig. 6

A3: Associations include atherosclerosis and its causes and hypercoagulable states. The blood pressure should be measured as hypertension is the most common systemic association. A complete blood count, ESR and plasma lipid and glucose levels are the minimum investigations routinely performed. In young patients and other situations with unusual features, more extensive investigation is indicated. Prophylactic low dose aspirin is usually prescribed following a retinal vein occlusion.

A4: Important complications of retinal venous occlusion include macular oedema with permanent visual loss and retinal and iris neovascularisation which may progress to rubeotic glaucoma. Retinal laser is sometimes indicated to treat neovascularisation and macular oedema.

SCENARIO 2

A5: The optic disc is swollen and pale. Anterior ischaemic optic neuropathy (AION) is very likely: the acute onset, the severity of the visual loss, the pallid quality of the optic disc swelling, the patient's age and the arteriopathic history. AION commonly causes an 'altitudinal' field loss in which the upper or lower half of the uniocular field is affected. Optic disc swelling is often predominantly superior or inferior. In a young patient, optic neuritis would be more likely, although this usually causes pain exacerbated by eye movement. Other causes of optic disc swelling are much less likely.

A6: These symptoms are typical of temporal (giant cell) arteritis. There may be tenderness along the superficial temporal arteries which may be thickened, nodular and non-pulsatile. In all cases of suspected or confirmed AION or central retinal arterial occlusion, you should ask about symptoms of giant cell arteritis and order an ESR (urgently) and a C-reactive protein level. A positive temporal artery biopsy finding is pathognomonic, but neither a low ESR nor a negative biopsy exclude the diagnosis.

A7: If you think that AION is due to giant cell arteritis, systemic steroids should be started immediately. This does not affect the result of any subsequent temporal artery biopsy but will lower an elevated C-reactive protein.

SCENARIO 3

A8: The Amsler grid shows a large positive scotoma at fixation, which almost always indicates a macular lesion. In an elderly patient, a history of rapidly progressive central distortion with preserved peripheral vision is highly suggestive of age-related macular degeneration with a choroidal neovascular membrane (CNVM). A large part of the macula in the right eye is affected by a combination of serous exudation and haemorrhage.

A9: Fundus fluorescein angiography (FFA) helps to confirm the diagnosis and may identify those uncommon cases which are suitable for photodynamic therapy (PDT).

A10: About half of all patients suffer the same problem in the fellow eye within 5 years. If any distortion occurs in the fellow eye, the patient should have an ophthalmic examination immediately to detect a lesion amenable to treatment.

Sudden visual loss

■ Most cases are due to obstruction of the venous or arterial circulation of the retina or optic nerve.

■ Retinal vein and artery occlusion produce characteristic and distinct retinal appearances; assess systemic vascular risk factors (hypertension, diabetes mellitus, atherosclerosis).

■ Anterior ischaemic optic neuropathy (AION) commonly features an 'altitudinal' field defect and a pale swollen optic disc; exclude temporal arteritis.

■ Exudative ('wet') age related macular degeneration: central vision loss, often with distortion; preservation of peripheral vision; early photodynamic therapy is sometimes indicated.

The acute red eye

A 48-year-old woman attended a hospital accident and emergency department. For the previous two days, her left eye had been inflamed and watering. There was slight blurring of vision and the eye was moderately uncomfortable. There was no history of trauma. The right eye was asymptomatic. There was no past eye history. She was fit and well and not taking any medication. The emergency physician diagnosed viral conjunctivitis and commenced a broad-spectrum topical antibiotic, arranging a routine review appointment in three days but warning the patient to return urgently prior to this if the symptoms worsened.

Q1: The acute red eye is a common ophthalmological presentation caused by conditions ranging from the trivial to the sight-threatening. List at least six important causes.

SCENARIO 1

The patient returned to hospital later the same day complaining that the pain in the left eye had become severe. There was now frontal headache and malaise. The vision in this eye had become much worse ('counting fingers' only). The eye was very inflamed and the cornea looked hazy (Fig. 1). The pupil was oval in shape and failed to react to either direct or consensual light stimulation. There was a left relative afferent pupillary defect.

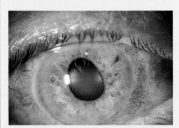

Fig. 1

Q2: What is the most likely diagnosis?

Q3: What features of the history and examination lead you to this conclusion?

Q4: What are the chief diagnostic alternatives and why?

Q5: How would you manage this patient?

SCENARIO 2

The patient attended the review appointment as planned. The left eye was feeling more comfortable and was less red, but the right eye was now suffering the same symptoms. Visual acuity was 6/6 in each eye, and pupil reactions were normal. The conjunctiva in both eyes was diffusely hyperaemic and there was a profuse watery discharge. There was no corneal haze.

Q6: The diagnosis is viral conjunctivitis. What features suggest that the cause is not a sight-threatening condition?

Q7: What is shown here (Fig. 2)?

Q8: What should you do about this (Fig. 2)?

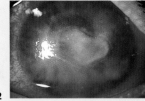

Fig. 2

Q9: What is shown here (Fig. 3)?

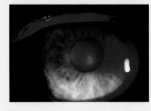

Fig.3

Q10: How do you manage this?

SCENARIO 3

The patient attended the next appointment as scheduled, but the left eye was now considerably more uncomfortable and visual acuity was reduced to 6/18. Photophobia (sensitivity to bright light) was a prominent feature. The emergency physician suspected acute glaucoma. The appearance of the left eye is shown in Figure 4.

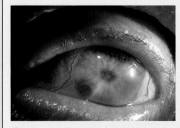

Fig. 4

Q11: Describe the abnormalities shown here and suggest the diagnosis.

Q12: What is the management of this condition?

Q13: Name six systemic associations of this disorder.

A1: Important causes of red eye include:

- conjunctivitis: infections (bacterial, viral), allergic, with blepharitis
- acute angle closure glaucoma
- acute iritis
- trauma: subconjunctival haemorrhage, corneal abrasion, corneal foreign body, penetrating injury
- keratitis: infections (herpetic, bacterial), marginal keratitis
- episcleritis
- scleritis
- subconjunctival haemorrhage: spontaneous or traumatic.

Condition		Configuration	Reactivity
Acute angle closure glaucoma	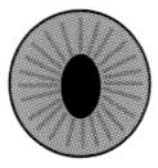	Mid-dilated, oval	Fixed to direct and consensual light stimulation ± RAPD
Acute iritis	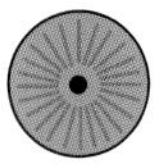	May be normal; often miotic due to iris spasm ± posterior synechiae	Normal or decreased reaction to direct and consensual light; no RAPD
Conjunctivitis	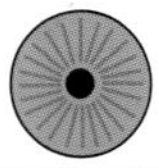	Normal in uncomplicated conjunctivitis [the majority]	Normal

Fig. 5 Pupillary signs in the acute red eye.

SCENARIO 1

A2: Acute glaucoma.

A3: Unilateral eye pain, often with headache, poor vision, a hazy cornea (due to oedema) and a oval mid-dilated fixed pupil are all typical of acute angle closure glaucoma. Patients may also describe haloes around lights as a result of the corneal oedema.

A4: Iritis is the main differential diagnosis, but few other conditions cause such pain with visual loss. Conjunctivitis and blepharitis cause discomfort only. Acute corneal problems may cause pain but usually there is a history of trauma or an obvious ulcer on staining with fluorescein.

A5: Urgent referral to an ophthalmologist is necessary, as permanent visual loss can rapidly occur if acute glaucoma is not treated promptly. The initial management is to lower the intraocular pressure using pilocarpine and systemic acetazolamide. Laser iridotomy is performed to prevent a further attack. The fellow eye must undergo prophylactic laser, as it is predisposed to an attack.

SCENARIO 2

A6: The visual acuities are good, although mild to moderate blurring may occur in conjunctivitis. A watery discharge with sticky lids in the morning is typical. The discharge of bacterial conjunctivitis is purulent, while that of allergic conjunctivitis is mucoid. The pupil reactions are normal (Fig. 5) and the corneas are clear.

A7: The photograph shows a corneal ulcer, probably bacterial in aetiology. This is a rare complication of simple conjunctivitis, but is more common in contact lens wearers. A simple corneal abrasion is clean, without corneal opacity. **You must always check the cornea when the eye is red.**

A8: Urgent ophthalmological referral is required.

A9: These are dendritic ulcers caused by the herpes simplex virus. A dendritic ulcer should not be treated with topical steroids, which will make it much worse. Again, this demonstrates the importance of a corneal examination when assessing the red eye.

A10: Topical aciclovir ointment is prescribed. Most cases resolve without significant scarring, but recurrence is common.

SCENARIO 3

A11: This is acute iritis. 'Ciliary injection' (conjunctival hyperaemia concentrated at the corneoscleral junction) is evident. The cornea appears slightly misty, but this is because of inflammatory cells and exudate in the anterior chamber and on the corneal endothelium. The pupil is constricted due to spasm; sometimes it is irregular. In iritis, inflammation is confined to the eyeball.

A12: Topical steroids are the main treatment. A dilating drop such as cyclopentolate or homatropine is also prescribed: this eases the pain and helps stop the formation of permanent posterior synechiae (adhesions between the iris and the lens).

A13: Three-quarters of all cases are idiopathic. Ankylosing spondylitis, Reiter's syndrome and other sero-negative arthritides, sarcoidosis, inflammatory bowel disease and, in children, juvenile chronic arthritis are the most frequently identified associations.

The acute red eye

- Significant visual loss and abnormal pupil reactions are key clues in the identification of serious disease.
- Acute angle closure glaucoma typically causes severe pain and redness, with greatly reduced vision, a hazy cornea and a fixed, mid-dilated pupil.
- Conjunctivitis causes mild blurring only, due to the accumulation of discharge; the corneas are clear and the pupils are normal.
- Acute iritis causes varying degrees of pain, photophobia and blurred vision; 'ciliary injection' is typical and the pupil is often small.

Trauma

A vagrant is brought into a hospital emergency department late at night.
He has been assaulted.

SCENARIO 1

He is not able to give a useful history other than that his right eye is sore and blurred.

Q1: What should you do?

Q2: What is shown here (Fig. 1)?

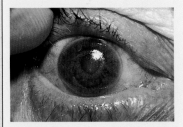

Fig. 1

Q3: What is the management?

Q4: What is the long-term outcome?

SCENARIO 2

He is not able to give a clear history, but remembers being punched and kicked in the face and reports that he can see very little with his right eye, the lids of which are beginning to swell greatly.

Q5: What is shown here (Fig. 2)?

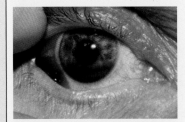

Fig. 2

Q6: What other ocular damage might have occurred?

Q7: What is the management of the condition shown in Figure 2?

Q8: What are the clinical features of an orbital blow-out fracture?

SCENARIO 3

There are multiple facial lacerations, some of which contain fragments of glass. It seems that he has been struck with a bottle. There is almost no sight at all in the right eye.

Q9: What is shown here (Fig. 3)?

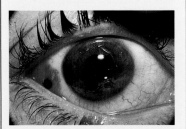

Fig. 3

Q10: What management is required?

Q11: What are the chief long-term consequences of this injury?

SCENARIO 1

A1:
- Try to quantify vision.
- Examine with a pen torch or at the slit lamp.
- Instil fluorescein and examine with a blue light.

A2: Fluorescein has been instilled and is staining a large central corneal abrasion.

A3: The conventional treatment is:
- chloramphenicol ointment
- a dilating drop, such as cyclopentolate or homatropine, which helps to reduce discomfort
- an occlusive dressing (a pad).

Daily or alternate day review is recommended until the abrasion has healed.

A4: Most corneal abrasions heal rapidly without any lasting effects. Occasionally corneal infection (keratitis) may occur, particularly if the injury is dirty or if a foreign body is present. Keratitis requires aggressive antibiotic treatment. The recurrent corneal erosion (abrasion) syndrome, in which attachment of the epithelium to its basement membrane is weak, can also ensue. It causes episodic symptoms of recurrent pain and watering, especially in the morning. Between attacks there is usually nothing to be seen on pen torch examination, though there may be punctate fluorescein staining. Management consists of regular lubrication, using artificial tear drops during the day and an ointment at night. Eventually there is spontaneous resolution. Occasionally there is an actual abrasion, which should be treated appropriately.

SCENARIO 2

A5: There is a subconjunctival haemorrhage together with a large hyphaema.

A6: Hyphaema, bleeding from the iris, indicates that the eye has suffered major trauma. Any other ocular structure might also be damaged. Chief problems are:

- corneal abrasion
- acute and chronic glaucoma
- cataract
- vitreous haemorrhage
- retinal damage: commotio (traumatic oedema); choroidal rupture, usually near the optic disc; macular damage; retinal detachment
- orbital blow-out fracture.

A7: The hyphaema should be managed by rest and topical steroid drops. Patients are often admitted to hospital. Once the hyphaema has cleared, the eye should be examined carefully for other problems. Until then, the patient should be warned that there may be permanent sight-threatening damage.

A8: The clinical features of orbital blow-out fracture are:

- enophthalmos which may be masked in the short term by orbital haemorrhage
- altered facial sensation in the region of the infraorbital nerve (the cheek)
- reduced vertical ocular movement (up and down), causing vertical double vision.

There is only rarely a fracture of the orbital rim, so palpation is unhelpful. Facial X-ray may help to confirm the diagnosis, but the definitive investigation is a CT scan.

SCENARIO 3

A9: There is a hint of hyphaema. The pupil and iris are distorted. The eye has been perforated across the cornea. There is a scleral haemorrhage, suggesting further perforation here also.

A10: You should suspect the presence of an intraocular foreign body. Clinical examination alone is unlikely to exclude this possibility, since there is so much hyphaema. Plain X-ray, ocular ultrasound and CT scan may be necessary. There is a significant risk of endophthalmitis (intraocular infection). The perforation must be repaired and antibiotic treatment administered.

A11: The important long-term consequences are:

- corneal scarring, causing astigmatism and opacity
- cataract
- retinal detachment
- glaucoma
- sympathetic ophthalmitis

The consequences of corneal scarring are most severe when located centrally, but peripheral scarring can cause significant astigmatism. Glaucoma may be severe and resistant to standard treatments. Sympathetic ophthalmitis, a severe form of uveitis occurring in the fellow eye, is a rare but serious complication of perforating trauma. It may be prevented by early removal of the damaged eye, so a careful assessment of the visual prognosis is crucial.

Trauma

- Assessment of visual function is essential in all cases of trauma.
- Corneal abrasion is common and heals rapidly with antibiotic ointment and padding.
- Hyphaema indicates severe eye trauma and is often accompanied by damage to other structures.
- A history of sharp trauma should raise the possibility of ocular perforation and even intraocular foreign body.

The squinting child

A four-year-old child is brought to clinic by her mother who has noticed a 'turn' in the left eye.

Q1: What are the key parts of the assessment of such a child?

SCENARIO 1

Q2: What does this show (Fig. 1)?

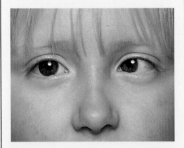

Fig. 1

The strabismus is of recent onset and there is a family history. Visual acuity (Sheridan–Gardiner testing) is 6/6 right, 6/24 left. The left eye is convergent, slowly taking up fixation when the right eye is covered. The retina is easily seen and is normal. Refraction shows that both eyes are hypermetropic, the left more so than the right.

Q3: What is the term used to describe the vision in the left eye?

Q4: What different types of refractive error are there and how are they corrected?

Q5: What is the appropriate management?

Q6: Should surgery be performed to straighten the eyes?

SCENARIO 2

The strabismus has come on very suddenly, and has caused the child to become distressed. Visual acuity (Sheridan–Gardiner testing) is right 6/6, left worse than 6/60. There is no refractive error.

Q7: What does this suggest and what should you do next?

Attempted ophthalmoscopy reveals a whitish lesion obstructing visualisation of the retina through the pupil.

Q8: What are the possible causes of this scenario?

Q9: What does this show (Fig. 2)?

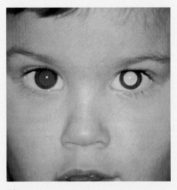

Fig. 2

Q10: What should you do if the child shown in Figure 2 presents to you?

Q11: What is the long-term prognosis for the conditions considered above?

SCENARIO 3

The child has been unwell and vomiting. She has been unsteady on her feet. Your cover test confirms there is a left convergent strabismus.

Q12: What does this test of ocular movement show (Fig. 3)?

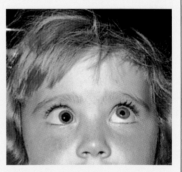

Fig. 3

Q13: What is the implication?

Q14: What should you do now?

A1: Assessment should include:
- measurement of visual acuity and binocular visual function (including 3-D vision)
- cover test for strabismus
- assessment of ocular movement
- measurement of refractive error
- retinal examination through dilated pupils.

SCENARIO 1

A2: There is a left convergent strabismus (esotropia).

A3: Amblyopia. The eye is structurally normal.

A4:
- Myopia (short sight): concave lens.
- Hypermetropia (long sight): convex lens.
- Astigmatism: requires a complex lens.
- Anisometropia: the refractive error differs significantly between the two eyes.

This child is both hypermetropic and anisometropic, which make amblyopia and strabismus very likely.

A5: Spectacles should be prescribed and worn full time. The right eye should be occluded in order to force the left eye to fixate. Amblyopia can be reversed by such treatment during the sensitive period of visual development, which ends at about 8 years of age.

A6: Surgery can change the angle of squint deviation, but it cannot reduce the refractive error or reverse the amblyopia, though parents often expect such outcomes. Treatment with spectacles and occlusion may straighten the eyes and reverse the amblyopia. Once the best possible result has been achieved, surgery to reduce any remaining angle of deviation may be performed for cosmetic reasons.

SCENARIO 2

A7: As there is no refractive error, you should suspect that more sinister pathology, not simple amblyopia, is causing the poor vision. You must dilate the pupil and examine the retina.

A8: The possible causes include:

- Retinoblastoma: a malignant tumour of the retina which is sometimes inherited (in which case it may be bilateral).
- Cataract: this will obscure the view of the retina. The degree of opacity is variable and may be unilateral or bilateral.
- Toxocara and toxoplasma: toxocara infection is usually acquired in infancy whereas toxoplasmosis is generally contracted in utero. Both can damage the macula.
- Persistence of embryological vitreous (persistent hyperplastic primary vitreous, or PHPV).

A9: Cataract.

A10: Refer the child immediately for an ophthalmological opinion.

A11: Death from retinoblastoma can be prevented with aggressive treatment, but sight cannot be saved and there is a long-term risk of a second malignancy in another tissue at a different site (e.g. a sarcoma).

The outcome of cataract surgery is unpredictable. In unilateral cataract there may be profound amblyopia which cannot be reversed. The visual outcome in bilateral cataract may be better. The major management problem is the correction of paediatric aphakia. Glasses may not be satisfactory, contact lenses may not be tolerated or may fall out and lens implants do not yet have an established role.
Visual loss from toxocara and toxoplasma is permanent. Toxoplasma retinitis may be recurrent over many years.
Mild PHPV can be removed by vitrectomy; PHPV is anyway unilateral.

SCENARIO 3

A12: The left eye fails to abduct (turn laterally), suggesting a lateral rectus palsy.

A13: A sixth nerve palsy is a likely cause, particularly since the child has other presenting problems. Suspect an intracranial cause. There may be disease directly affecting the sixth nerve, or the paresis may be a 'false localising sign' of raised intracranial pressure.

A14: Refer the child to a paediatrician urgently.

The squinting child

- Most paediatric strabismus is associated with a refractive error.
- Assess visual function: amblyopia is common.
- Exclude intraocular pathology (look for leukocoria).
- Ensure eye movements are full: beware a sixth nerve palsy.

'Spots before the eyes'

A 63-year-old male attended his optometrist complaining of 'spots before the eyes'. This phrase is commonly used by patients to describe two distinct types of symptom:

- 'scintillating scotomata' – often compared to the distorting effect of water running down a window, a kaleidoscope pattern or zig-zag lines;
- 'floaters' – an exaggeration of the physiological phenomenon seen when staring into the distance against a pale background such as the sky.

Q1: Suggest causes of these two types of symptom.

SCENARIO 1

The man reported the presence of several mobile translucent strands and specks, 'like a cobweb', and a flickering light in the left eye for three or four days. There was no history of trauma.

Q2: The patient is myopic. Why is this important?

Q3: The visual acuity was 6/6 in each eye. Does this provide reassurance that a sight-threatening condition is not present?

Q4: What is the significance of the flickering light?

Q5: What simple examination techniques should you perform?

SCENARIO 2

The patient described three or four episodes a week of visual disturbance lasting ten minutes which affected the left half of the field of vision in both eyes. He compared the appearance to that of multiple streaks of lightning. Although he had been aware of the symptom for four or five years, the frequency had recently increased.

Q6: What other clinical features should you ask about?

Q7: Besides the eyes, what aspects of a physical examination are important?

Q8: This abnormality was identified on retinal examination (Fig. 1). What is it and how will it alter your management?

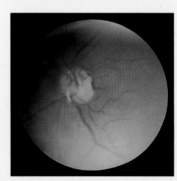

Fig. 1

SCENARIO 3

Vision in the left eye was moderately blurred immediately after waking up in the morning, clearing over the course of the day but with persistence of floating blobs and streaks. Visual acuities were 6/12 right, 6/36 left. There was no relative afferent pupillary defect.

Q9: What physical sign is demonstrated here (Fig. 2)?

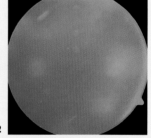

Fig. 2

Q10: This is the retina of the asymptomatic fellow eye (Fig. 3). What does it show? Can you make a connection between the symptoms and signs of the two eyes? What treatment is required?

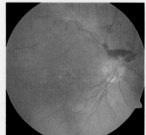

Fig. 3

Q11: What else might cause the signs seen in the left eye?

A1: 'Scintillating scotomata' are usually associated with an episode of underperfusion of the retina or cerebral cortex. Migraine is common; emboli and giant cell arteritis should also be considered.

'Floaters' or terms such as a cobweb, a fly, a net curtain, a tadpole or a hair are frequently used by patients to describe the appearance of mobile opacities within the vitreous body. Typical causes are:

- vitreous degeneration and posterior vitreous detachment
- vitreous haemorrhage
- posterior segment inflammation (uveitis).

SCENARIO 1

A2: The major diagnostic possibilities are retinal detachment and posterior vitreous detachment (with or without a retinal tear). Myopia is associated with both of these.

A3: The visual acuity in an eye with a retinal detachment will be affected only if the central macula is detached. Good vision is therefore falsely reassuring. In fact, retinal detachment that has not yet progressed to involve the macula carries a better prognosis if surgical reattachment is successful.

A4: When a posterior vitreous detachment occurs, the collapsing vitreous gel may exert traction on the retina, stimulating the retina so that it 'sees' a flickering light. This traction may tear the retina. However, the symptom can be present without a retinal break, and conversely a break can be present without the symptom.

A5: You can test the peripheral field of vision using your fingers. In the presence of a retinal detachment, this may reveal a scotoma. Use your ophthalmoscope to look at the retinal periphery: even with the pupil undilated, you may see a grey area suggesting a retinal detachment.

It is unlikely that you will identify a retinal break and you may never see a retinal detachment. Sudden onset of floaters and a flashing light should alert you to refer your patient for ophthalmic examination.

SCENARIO 2

A6: The most likely diagnosis is migraine, though an embolic or other vascular cause should be considered. Important features to ask about include:

- The duration of each episode: typically 5–20 minutes in migraine.
- Headache: migrainous pain is throbbing, often unilateral and often follows the visual symptoms. However, headache is not necessary for diagnosis ('acephalgic' migraine).
- A past or family history of migraine.
- Other neurological symptoms.
- Vascular risk factors include diabetes mellitus, ischaemic heart disease, peripheral vascular disease, hypertension, hyperlipidaemia, smoking, polycythaemia, arteritis.

In a young patient with a typical history of migraine, investigation beyond a careful history and examination is usually unnecessary. Persistent deficits require further investigation.

A7: Neurological and cardiovascular examination.

A8: This is an embolus in a retinal arteriole. It is likely to have arisen in a carotid artery on the same side, causing uniocular symptoms. Emboli involving the posterior cerebral circulation usually cause binocular symptoms. Investigation for vascular risk factors and for the presence of an embolic source is necessary. Specific preventative treatment may be indicated.

SCENARIO 3

A9: This is a diffusely dimmed red reflex. To examine the red reflex shine the light from a direct ophthalmoscope into the eye from about half a metre away and observe the pupil through the eyepiece. Opacities in the usually clear ocular media such as cataract and vitreous haemorrhage will be apparent. Vitreous opacities appear to bounce or wobble as the eye moves. In this case the patient has vitreous opacities due to a vitreous haemorrhage.

A10: This is proliferative retinopathy, in this case due to diabetes mellitus. The left eye has suffered a vitreous haemorrhage, so presumably the left eye also has new vessels. The right eye, which sees normally because there has been no haemorrhage and because the macula is not affected, requires urgent retinal laser treatment. If the haemorrhage in the left eye does not clear rapidly to allow laser treatment, surgical removal of the vitreous should be considered.

A11: Most cases of vitreous haemorrhage occur in patients with diabetes mellitus. Other causes include retinal venous occlusion, exudative age-related macular degeneration and retinal artery macroaneurysms. Not infrequently, a spontaneous haemorrhage clears rapidly and a cause is never identified.

'Spots before the eyes'

- Floaters are most commonly due to vitreous degeneration or posterior vitreous detachment; a normal examination does not exclude a retinal tear which may progress to retinal detachment.
- Vitreous haemorrhage: examine the other eye; consider diabetes.
- Other visual phenomena
  - retinal or cerebral underperfusion
  - look for features of arteriopathy.
- Migraine
  - a variety of visual symptoms, unilateral headache, nausea
  - investigate atypical cases.

Irritable eyes

A 37-year-old woman was referred to an ophthalmologist by her GP. For more than two years she had endured progressively worsening grittiness and burning of both eyes, often associated with redness and watering. The symptoms were present on most days.

Q1: Suggest some possible causes.

SCENARIO 1

The patient reported that the symptoms were worse towards the end of the day, particularly in a warm dry environment. The GP had provisionally diagnosed dry eyes and prescribed artificial tears, with some benefit. The patient also complained of a persistently dry mouth.

Rheumatoid arthritis had been diagnosed a number of years previously.

Q2: Based on the history, is the GP's diagnosis likely to be correct?

Q3: What simple examination techniques might be used to confirm the presence of dry eyes?

Q4: Suggest a modified treatment regimen.

SCENARIO 2

The patient's major complaint was itching. The discomfort was worse in spring than at other times of the year. She had suffered from asthma as a child, and moderate to severe eczema throughout her life. There was a family history of atopy.
The eyelid skin was red and excoriated, and there was a stringy mucous discharge. Eversion of the upper eyelids revealed large conjunctival papillae (Fig. 1). There was superior corneal scarring.

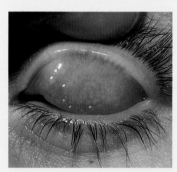

Fig. 1

Q5: What is the diagnosis?

Q6: What are the chief complications of this condition?

Q7: Suggest appropriate treatment.

SCENARIO 3

The symptoms of grittiness, burning and redness were worse on waking in the morning, when there was frequently mild stickiness or crusting of the lids.

Q8: Describe the abnormalities shown here (Fig. 2) and suggest the diagnosis.

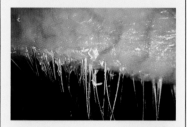

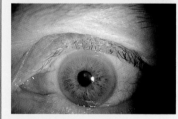

Fig. 2

Q9: What treatment is appropriate?

Q10: What skin condition is shown here (Fig. 3) and how is it related to the answer to Q8?

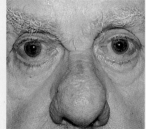

Fig. 3

A1: Common causes of chronic irritable eyes include:

- blepharitis
- dry eyes
- allergic conjunctivitis
- aberrant eyelash growth (trichiasis)
- entropion, ectropion
- refractory infective conjunctivitis (e.g. Chlamydia)
- thyroid eye disease
- contact lens intolerance
- sensitivity to long-term topical medications.

SCENARIO 1

A2: The patient almost certainly has dry eyes, which is a common ocular complication of rheumatoid arthritis. Oral dryness was also present, suggesting 'secondary Sjögren's syndrome'. The associated watering is 'paradoxical': the irritation causes reflex lacrimation so dry eye may still be present.

A3: Tear film quantity: Schirmer's test measures the production of tears, and the height of the tear meniscus can be measured at the slit lamp. Tear film quality is also important: look for the break-up time of the tear film after instillation of fluorescein. There may also be punctate staining of the inferior third of the cornea and strands of mucus.

A4: Reduce tear film evaporation: humidify dry rooms and fit side guards to spectacles to reduce air flow across the corneas. A variety of tear substitutes are available (drops, gels and ointments). The patient should be encouraged to experiment to determine personal preference. Ointment blurs the vision, so it is generally used at night only. Many patients are sensitive to the preservatives in drops: preservative-free preparations are available but are much more expensive. Artificial tears rapidly clear from the eye, so that in severe dry eye, drops may have to be given very frequently. Lacrimal punctal occlusion can be considered if topical treatment is insufficient. Patients with arthritic hands may be unable to handle standard dropper bottles.

SCENARIO 2

A5: The diagnosis is atopic keratoconjunctivitis, a chronic form of allergic conjunctivitis. It is most commonly seen in young males with a history and/or a family history of atopy.

A6: This is a potentially sight-threatening condition which can be difficult to control. Complications include corneal ulceration and scarring, keratoconus and cataract.

A7: Known allergens should be avoided where possible. Topical mast cell stabilisers (sodium cromoglicate, lodoxamide and nedocromil) are the chief treatment. Topical vasoconstrictor/antihistamine combinations and the topical antihistamines levocabastine and azelastine give short-term but immediate relief of itching. Systemic antihistamines may also be helpful. Moderate to severe cases require topical steroids, preferably for short courses only. Long-term steroid use carries the risk of secondary cataract and glaucoma.

SCENARIO 3

A8: The eyelid skin is thickened and inflamed, especially at the lid margins. There is crusting and scaling around the lashes and a small amount of mucopurulent discharge at the medial canthus. Mild conjunctival hyperaemia is evident. The patient has severe blepharitis: a chronic inflammation of the eyelids with an infective element. Complications, usually seen in severe cases only, include corneal ulceration at the limbus (marginal keratitis) and scarring.

A9: The mainstay of treatment is a daily eyelid 'hygiene' routine to reduce debris and bacterial load. Long-term antibiotic ointment can be useful, applied to the eyelid margins once or twice daily. Inadequate tear production may co-exist and it is important to treat this adequately. The condition is chronic and relapsing, but adequate relief of symptoms can usually be achieved by these simple measures. If symptoms persist, a course of low dose oral tetracycline (or erythromycin) for 6–12 weeks may be prescribed.

A10: This is acne rosacea, a skin condition manifesting with telangiectases, papules and pustules on the facial skin. (There are no comedones, unlike acne vulgaris). Severe blepharitis and blepharoconjunctivitis are common in patients with acne rosacea, and corneal complications are more frequent and more severe.

Irritable eyes

- Chronic or recurrent moderate ocular discomfort can be very distressing.
- A dry eye state causes grittiness and paradoxical watering.
- The clinical features of allergic conjunctivitis include itching, stringy white mucus and large conjunctival papillae; most patients have a history of other atopic disease.
- Blepharitis:
    - symptoms are often much worse than the signs so it can easily be overlooked.
    - scaling and crusting of the eyelashes
    - morning stickiness
    - associated with acne rosacea
    - treatment: regular lid hygiene, antibiotic ointment, tear replacements, systemic tetracycline or erythromycin.

Double vision

A 58-year-old man attended his family doctor. Two days previously he had become aware of horizontal double vision. The images were most widely separated on gaze to the right. Covering either eye caused one image to disappear. There was no significant past medical or ophthalmic history. The general practitioner contacted an ophthalmologist, who saw the patient urgently.

Q1: Most double vision in adults is caused by incomitant squint due to neurological or muscular dysfunction, or to mechanical restriction of the eye muscles. Using these headings, list some causes.

SCENARIO 1

Cover testing in the primary position showed a moderate right convergent squint, worse for distance than near. There was limitation of abduction of the right eye (Fig. 1). The eyes were otherwise normal, as was a general neurological examination.

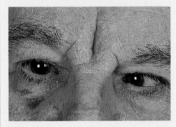

Fig. 1

Q2: Which muscle is affected and what is its nerve supply?

Q3: How might temporary control of the double vision be achieved?

Q4: What investigations are necessary?

Q5: What is the likely outcome for the double vision?

SCENARIO 2

There were some additional symptoms: the eyes had been red and irritable for some months and had assumed a 'staring' appearance (Fig. 2).

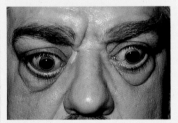

Fig. 2

Q6: What further information would you like to know?

Q7: Why is there double vision?

Q8: Sight loss is a rare but preventable complication. How might it occur?

Q9: List some simple tests of visual function you can perform to identify such a complication.

SCENARIO 3

By late afternoon when the patient attended the ophthalmology clinic the symptoms had worsened, with double vision now present on left gaze also. He described how his eyelids tended to droop towards the end of the day, especially if he was tired. Cover testing demonstrated an alternating divergent squint. There was 2 mm of ptosis bilaterally, and sustained upgaze for one minute caused this to increase.

Q10: What is the likely cause and what pharmacological test is indicated?

Q11: What blood test is indicated?

Q12: What is this (Fig. 3)? What other ocular features would you suspect?

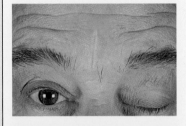

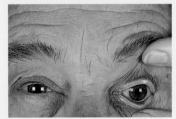

Fig. 3

A1: Causes of incomitant squint include:

- neurological – paresis of nerve supply to extraocular muscles (III, IV, VI), central nervous system disease (e.g. internuclear ophthalmoplegia)
- muscular – myasthenia gravis
- mechanical restriction – thyroid eye disease, orbital wall fracture, orbital tumour or 'pseudotumour'.

Other causes of double vision include surgical overcorrection of squint, decompensation of a latent squint, and problems with spectacles (correction or fit). Disorders of the cornea or lens (keratoconus, cataract, lens dislocation) can cause monocular diplopia (persists when unaffected eye is covered).

SCENARIO 1

A2: The muscle is the right lateral rectus which is supplied by the sixth cranial nerve.

A3: An occlusive patch over one eye will immediately eliminate the double vision. A temporary plastic prism applied to the patient's own spectacle lens is effective and cosmetically more acceptable. It will need to be replaced as the angle of the strabismus changes.

A4: Since most cranial nerve palsies are associated with atherosclerosis, a vascular work-up is necessary. Progression of a palsy, involvement of other nerves or additional symptoms (especially neurological) should lead you to suspect a more sinister cause and investigate accordingly. Most cases of paresis of the oculomotor (third) nerve, including all of those with pupil involvement, require urgent assessment to exclude an intracranial aneurysm.

A5: Spontaneous recovery is the rule, over a period of up to 6 months.

SCENARIO 2

A6: You should suspect dysthyroid eye disease. Although this can occur in the absence of thyroid gland dysfunction, most patients are thyrotoxic. You should ask about weight and appetite, heat tolerance, tremor, palpitations, etc. Thyroid function testing is required.

A7: The extraocular muscles are infiltrated with inflammatory cells and oedema, causing mechanical restriction and weakness. Involvement of a combination of muscles of the two eyes may produce a complicated pattern of eye movement with double vision in many positions of gaze. However inferior rectus muscle is often the first to be involved, causing vertical double vision.

A8: Optic nerve compression is the chief cause (Fig. 4). Proptosis leading to corneal exposure and ulceration may also occur.

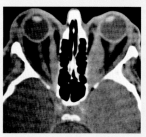

Fig. 4

A9: Simple tests of optic nerve function:

- visual acuity (using a standard or reduced Snellen chart)
- comparison of colour appreciation between the two eyes (red pen top or Ishihara plates)
- pupil tests (for the presence of a relative afferent pupillary defect)
- assessment of the visual fields to confrontation.

In the early stages the optic disc may be swollen; later, optic atrophy may ensue. Acute optic nerve compression in thyroid eye disease requires immediate treatment. Options include systemic steroids, local radiotherapy and surgical decompression.

SCENARIO 3

A10: The clinical findings strongly suggest myasthenia gravis, which can mimic cranial nerve palsies and thyroid eye disease. A Tensilon (edrophonium) test usually confirms the diagnosis.

A11: Acetylcholine receptor antibodies are present in the majority of patients with myasthenia gravis. Further investigation, often undertaken by a neurologist, includes imaging to detect a thymoma, together with additional immunological studies.

A12: This is a third nerve palsy, another important cause of a ptosis with double vision, though the ptosis will usually mask the diplopia. The eye is abducted as sixth nerve innervation is intact. The pupil may be dilated.

Double vision

- Most diplopia occurs in adults and is caused by incomitant squint due to isolated palsy of third, fourth or sixth cranial nerves.
- Thyroid eye disease: usually gradual onset, inferior and medial rectus involvement, other ocular and systemic features.
- Myasthenia gravis may mimic other motility abnormalities; ptosis is common.
- Ptosis: 3rd nerve palsy (dilated pupil, abducted eye); Horner's syndrome (constricted pupil); age-related; trauma; myasthenia gravis.

Eye database (UK perspective)

EyeUK
www.eyeuk.com
EyeUK is an index of UK websites related to the eye, vision and ophthalmology.

Medmark Ophthalmology sub-category
www.medmark.org/oph
Provides a similar service to EyeUK, but indexes sites worldwide.

Action for Blind People
www.afbp.org

Albinism Fellowship
www.albinism.org.uk
Albinism Fellowship provides advice and support for people with an interest in albinism and a range of appropriate services that provide information, raise awareness, challenge misrepresentation, improve self-esteem and give opportunities to meet other people affected by the condition.

American Academy of Ophthalmology see EyeNet

American Academy of Optometry
www.aaopt.org

American Academy of Optometry – British Chapter
www.academy.org.uk
The aims of the Chapter are to promote excellence in the practise of optometry.

Association of Blind Piano Tuners
www.uk-piano.org/abpt
The Association of Blind Piano Tuners exists to serve the professional and particular needs of its members and other blind and partially sighted piano tuners throughout the world.

Association for Research in Vision and Ophthalmology
www.arvo.org
The website of the Association for Research in Vision and Ophthalmology contains searchable databases of abstracts accepted for previous and up coming ARVO conferences.

Association of Vision Science Librarians
spectacle.berkeley.edu/~library/AVSL.HTM

Blackburn and District Blind Society
www.blackburnblind.org.uk
A registered charity catering for both visually impaired and blind people. It covers all ages from babies and toddlers to adults. It offers a full range of services and facilities for everyone.

Blindcare
www.btinternet.com/~blindcare

The Blind Youth Group
www.tbyg.co.uk
Blackburn-based group of blind and visually impaired teenagers who meet up once a month to arrange outings and fundraising events.

Brighton Society for the Blind, Brighton, UK
www.bsblind.co.uk

British Blind Sport
www.britishblindsport.org.uk
BBS is a charity that provides sporting opportunities for blind and partially sighted people. Members take part in a variety of sports, and activites range from amateur 'have a go' days to competing in international events.

British Computer Association of the Blind
www.bcab.org.uk

British Diabetic Association
www.diabetes.org.uk

British Journal of Ophthalmology
bjo.bmjjournals.com

British Ophthalmic Anaesthesia Society
www.boas.org

British Ophthalmic Photographic Association
www.bopa.org.uk

British Retinitis Pigmentosa Society
www.brps.demon.co.uk
The BRPS was founded in 1975 and is a registered charity set up for the benefit of those with RP. It is a self-help group that seeks to help its members live with and overcome their visual problems and to bring relief by stimulating research into the causes and eventually the treatment of RP. This is achieved by funding a range of research projects using money raised, mainly through its branches, for this purpose.

British Wireless for the Blind Fund
www.blind.org.uk
The BWBF provides, on a permanent free loan basis, radios, radio cassette recorders and CD radio cassette recorders, to UK registered blind people, over the age of 8 and who are in need.

Cancer of the Eye LinkLine (C.E.L.L.)
pages.zoom.co.uk/cell/index.htm
C.E.L.L. is a voluntary helpline that can offer support, information or a shoulder to lean on to anyone suffering from eye cancer or other eye trauma, or their friends or family.

Cardiff Institute for the Blind
www.cibi.co.uk/dsp_splash_flash.cfm

Church and Blindness
www.church4blind.org.uk

Cochrane Eyes and Vision Group
www.archie.ucl.ac.uk
Preparing, maintaining and promoting access to systematic reviews of interventions used to treat or prevent eye disease. The website contains information about published and ongoing reviews and ways to get involved.

County Durham Society for the Visually Handicapped
members.aol.com/cdsvh/cdsvh.htm

Cyngor Cymru i'r Deillion/Wales Council for the Blind
www.wcb-ccd.org.uk
CCD yw'r prif sefydliad yng Nghymru ym maes nam ar y
golwg, sy'n gweithio gyda rhwydwaith o asiantaethau
gwirfoddol a statudol i wella'r ddarpariaeth ar gyfer pobl a
phroblemau gyda'u golwg yng Nghymru.

Deafblind UK
www.deafblinduk.org.uk
Deafblind UK specialises in meeting the needs and
developing the potential of adults who are both deaf and
blind. A range of comprehensive services are available to
deafblind members, their support assistants and
professionals in this field. They include training in
communication and rehabilitation skills; a free 24-hour
helpline; a regional network of staff, support workers and
volunteers; a varied leisure programme and a range of
publications in large print, Braille, Moon and on audio-tape.

Department of Health, UK – Action on Cataracts – Guidance
on good practice
www.doh.gov.uk/cataracts

Department of Health, UK – Deafblind site
www.doh.gov.uk/scg/deafblind/index.htm

Division of Orthoptics, University of Liverpool
www.liv.ac.uk/~pcknox
Departmental website detailing the teaching and research of
staff in the academic Orthoptics Department at Liverpool.
Includes links to other vision and oculomotor websites.

Echurch-UK
www.echurch-uk.org/index.html _top
An email discussion group for visually impaired Christians.

Ectodermal Dysplasia Society
www.ectodermaldysplasia.org
The Ectodermal Dysplasia Society is a support group for
families affected by ED. It has grown from contact between
two families in 1984 to a group now representing over 100
affected families.

English Blind Golf Association
www.blindgolf.co.uk/index.php
The EBGA is a voluntarily run organization, which provides
quality competition and training in golf for registered blind
people throughout England and Wales.

European Ophthalmic Pathology Society
www.helsinki.fi/laak/silk/perus/modern/eopshome.htm

European Society of Cataract and Refractive Surgery
www.escrs.ie
The Society offers its members an opportunity to share their
knowledge and experience as eye surgeons and to exchange
views and information on the various techniques involved in
this fast developing sector of ophthalmology.

Experimental Ophthalmology Unit, Liverpool, UK
www.liv.ac.uk/ophthalmology
Centre for control and treatment of eye disorders – interests
include AMD, corneal scarring, diabetes, ED, genetics,
glaucoma, melanoma and PVR.

The Eye Book
www.eyeuk.com/eyebook
This book is for popular interest rather than being an academic
textbook. It is aimed at everyone who has glasses or needs
glasses, or anyone who has a relative with an eye complaint.
The book would be a first introduction to a student who is
considering a future in orthoptics or optometry, a nurse who
might specialise in eye care and a 'catch up' for a G.P.

EyeCancer
www.eyecancer.com
An educational website for patients with eye cancer and for
the healthcare professionals who treat them.

Eyeless Trust
www.eyeless.org.uk

EyeLibrary
www.eyelibrary.org
Mostly medical retina images and fluorescein angiograms.

EyeNet
www.eyenet.org/aao_index.html
The website of the American Academy of Ophthalmology
contains information on a wide range of issues of particular
interest to North American eyecare professionals.

EyesOnline
www.eyesonline.co.uk
An online, one-stop shop, for all information relating to the
eye, eye care and eye fashion. Has a large number of links to
manufacturers, opticians and other eye-related resources.

EyeText
http://www.eyetext.net
An ophthalmic resource site for (and restricted to) eyecare
professionals. It has three major sections of content: a
collection of monographs which will eventually form an
eTextbook, an interlinked set of editable ophthalmic notes
called 'iNotes' and an image database.

Fight for Sight
www.fightforsight.org.uk

Glaucoma Foundation
www.glaucoma-foundation.org
The website of the Glaucoma Foundation contains general
information about glaucoma including a list of risk factors for
the disease.

Global Medical Education and Training
www.gmet.net
A constantly updated resource of expert eye-related
information specifically designed to cater to the needs of
medical and paramedical professions.

Grafton Optical
www.graftonoptical.com

Grampian Society for the Blind
www.grampianblind.org
The Society is an independent charity providing social work,
rehabilitation and charitable services to 2500 visually impaired
people in Aberdeen, Aberdeenshire and Moray, Scotland.

Guide Dogs for the Blind Association
www.gdba.org.uk
The website of the Guide Dogs for the Blind Association contains information on its scheme for training guide dogs, plus information on its other activities which help improve the independence of those with a visual impairment.

Have Fun with Strabismus
www.xs4all.nl/~yskes/strab
This site offers an innovative insight into strabismus (i.e. the science of squints) and, as well as detailed background information, it includes images of celebrities with this condition.

The Health Centre UK – Eye Conditions and Visual Handicap
www.healthcentre.org.uk/hc/pages/eye.htm
The Health Centre is here to guide you through the huge amount of medical and health information from the UK that is available on the internet.

Henshaws Society for Blind People
www.hsbp.co.uk/index.htm

Herefordshire Disablement Information Advice Line
www.kc3.co.uk/dial
Herefordshire DIAL provides a free, impartial and confidential service of information, advice, and practical help to answer questions which can confront a person with a disability.

Institute of Ophthalmology
www.ucl.ac.uk/ioo

Interactive Eye
www.interactiveeye.com/home/index.asp
A scientific and educational resource for ophthalmologists, Interactive Eye allows users to submit content and share information. Have a look and start interacting!

International Glaucoma Association
www.iga.org.uk

The International Society for Eye Research
www.iser.org

Jubilee Sailing Trust
www.jst.org.uk
The JST enables able-bodied and physically disabled people to share the adventure of tall ship sailing. The JST owns tall ships Lord Nelson and Tenacious.

The Keratoconus Self Help and Support Group
www.keratoconus-group.org.uk

Lawson Large Print
www.largeprint.org
Teacher of the visually impaired modifies the Oxford Reading Tree, a reading programme for beginner readers. The stories are in large print and are fully illustrated.

LOOK – The National Federation of Families with Visually Impaired Children
www.look-uk.org

Macular Degeneration Network
www.macular-degeneration.org
An educational website for patients with macular degeneration and the health professionals who care for them.

Macular Disease Society
www.maculardisease.org

Marfan Association UK
www.marfan.org.uk/pages/html/home.htm

Medical Retina Group
www.medicalretina.org.uk
Information about the Medical Retina Group. An annual meeting is held every year as a satellite meeting of the Oxford Ophthalmological Congress.

Micro and Anophthalmic Children's Society
www.macs.org.uk

Moorfields Eye Hospital
www.moorfields.org.uk

National Library for the Blind
www.nlbuk.org
The National Library for the Blind is a free library service for visually impaired readers who want books in accessible formats. Books can be delivered or electronic files can be downloaded from this website.

North-East Rehabilitation Officers
www.nero-rehab.org.uk/

North of England Ophthalmological Society
www.neos.demon.co.uk

Nurses Eye Site
www.nurseseyesite.nhs.uk

OMNI – Ophthalmology Organising Medical Networked
omni.ac.uk/browse/mesh/detail/C0029087L0029087.html
Information is the UK gateway to quality biomedical and health information on the Internet, maintaining a searchable directory of reviews and links to quality Internet-accessible resources.

Ophtalmologiefr.com
www.ophtalmologiefr.com

Ophthalmic Research Network
www.site4sight.org.uk
The Ophthalmic Research Network is a web resource for all ophthalmologists and allied professions throughout the UK. All are free to post information.

Ophthalmology in Manchester
www.man.ac.uk/ophthalmology

Ophthalmology in Oxford
www.eye.ox.ac.uk/index.htm

Oxfordshire Association for the Blind
www.oxeyes.hiway.co.uk

Patient UK – Eye Health
www.patient.co.uk/showdoc.asp?doc=14

Retinitis Pigmentosa Site – Gordon Love
members.tripod.co.uk/lademill/rp.htm
This page gives a short personal account of one experience of retinitis pigmentosa (RP), together with the author's recommended scientific and related sites providing information on RP.

Royal Blind School, Edinburgh
www.royalblindschool.org.uk

Royal College of Ophthalmologists
www.rcophth.ac.uk

Royal London Society for the Blind
www.rlsb.org.uk

Royal National College for the Blind, Hereford
www.rncb.ac.uk
The UK's leading residential college for people who are blind or partially sighted. Providing a range of fulltime programmes and short courses designed to prepare people for progression to further education, university and the world of work, but most importantly, life.

Royal National Institute for the Blind
www.rnib.org.uk

Royal School for the Blind, Liverpool
www.rsblind.org.uk

Sense: The National Deaf Blind and Rubella Association
www.sense.org.uk
Sense is the national voluntary organisation supporting and campaigning for people who are deafblind, their families, their carers, and professionals who work with them. People of all ages and with widely varying conditions use Sense's specialist services.

Sheffield Royal Society for the Blind
www.srsb.org.uk _top
Local voluntary organisation providing a comprehensive range of services for visually impaired people in Sheffield.

Sight Savers International
www.sightsavers.org.uk
Sight Savers International is the UK's leading charity working to prevent and cure blindness in developing countries. During the last 50 years it has helped restore sight to over 4 million people and treated more than 45 million for sight threatening conditions.

SPecific Eye ConditionS (SPECS)
www.eyeconditions.org.uk _top
A not-for-profit umbrella group of patient groups for eye conditions and diseases.

St Vincent's School for Blind and Partially Sighted Children
www.stvin.org.uk

Success in MRCOphth
www.mrcophth.com
The first site in the UK devoted to passing MRCOphth/FRCS/MRCS with tips on clinical examination, multiple choice questions and picture diagnostic tests. Improve your chance of becoming a member of the Royal College of Ophthalmologists, United Kingdom.

Talking Newspaper Association of the UK
www.tnauk.org.uk
Provides newspapers and magazines in alternative formats to print for the visually impaired and disabled. It currently lists over 200 publications from around the world. Formats are audio cassettes, floppy disks, CD-ROM and e-text via e-mail.

UK Helplines for Visually Handicapped and Hearing Impaired
www.watb.net/info/h_lines/v_h_cap.shtml

Ulverscroft Group
www.edisure.com/~ulverscroft/uk/ukindex.html

University of Iowa's Department of Ophthalmology and Visual Sciences
webeye.ophth.uiowa.edu

VitreoRetinal Symposia
www.vrs-online.com
The VitreoRetinal Symposia (VRS) are a series of annual meetings featuring vitrectomy wetlabs and prominent international speakers who discuss the opportunities and limitations of selected vitreoretinal diagnostic and therapeutic approaches.

Visual Impairment North-East (VINE)
www.vine-simspecs.org.uk
VINE is a registered charity. VINE produces a regional directory of services available to the visually impaired, and also manufactures 'Simulation Spectacles'.

Visual Impairment Scotland
www.viscotland.org.uk

Wales Council for the Blind/Cyngor Cymru i'r Deillion
www.wcb-ccd.org.uk
WCB is the leading Welsh organisation in the field of visual impairment, working with a network of voluntary and statutory agencies to improve provision for people with sight problems in Wales.

The West of England School for Children with Little or No Sight
www.westengland.devon.sch.uk/index.htm
The South West's foremost specialist provision for young people who are visually impaired.

Yahoo (USA)
dir.yahoo.com/Health/Medicine/Ophthalmology

Yahoo UK and Ireland Ophthalmology sub-category
www.yahoo.co.uk/Health/Medicine/Ophthalmology
The Yahoo ophthalmology sub-category index contains comprehensive lists of links to ophthalmic related companies, conferences, institutes, journals, etc.

Index

Indexer: Dr Laurence Errington.